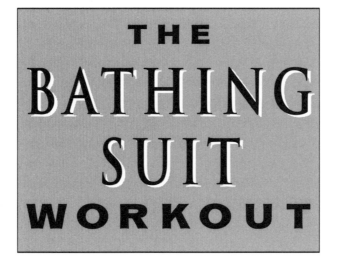

THE
BATHING
SUIT
WORKOUT

JOYCE L. VEDRAL, PH.D.

THE
BATHING
SUIT
WORKOUT

WARNER BOOKS

A Time Warner Company

Warner Books, Inc., 1271 Avenue of the Americas, New York, NY 10020
Visit our Web site at www.warnerbooks.com

 A Time Warner Company

Printed in the United States of America

ISBN 0-7394-0335-4

Cover design by Elaine Groh
Cover photo by Don Banks
Book design by Stanley Drate/ Folio Graphics Co., Inc.
Bodywear provided by Dance France, 1-800-421-1543
Photography by Don Banks
Gym shoes by Reebok International

To all of us,
the women who want
a bathing suit body—
whether or not
it's bathing suit season.

ACKNOWLEDGMENTS

To Jessica Papin, for your continual support and enthusiasm and for your kind willingness to go the extra mile.

To Mel Berger, my agent, for your cheerful wisdom.

To Diane Luger and Jacki Merri Meyer for your dedication to the cover art.

To Larry Kirshbaum, Mel Parker, and Emi Battaglia for being every author's dream when it comes to backing me up.

To Don Banks for your artistic photography.

Darriane, for your talent in hair design and makeup.

To Dance France for providing all of the workout clothing.

To Las Vegas Athletic Clubs in Las Vegas, Nevada, for providing a complete fitness facility (baby-sitting included) and to Chad and Karen Smith for your sensitivity and intelligence in management and personal attention.

To Joe and Betty Weider, who started it all!

To Rosa and Mike Tulane, true friends and enthusiastic supporters.

To you, the women who have written to me requesting such a book.

To Michelle, Kelley, Anita, Chris, and Ivonne for going the extra mile in your workouts.

CONTENTS

1   RECLAIM YOUR WAIST, HIPS, THIGHS, AND BUTT   1

2   THE SKINNY ON FAT!   9

3   BEFORE AND AFTER   23

4   WHAT YOU NEED TO KNOW, WHAT YOU NEED TO FORGET!   31

5   HOW TO DO THE BATHING SUIT WORKOUT   51

6   THE BATHING SUIT WORKOUT   63

7   THE BATHING SUIT DIET   127

8   EXTRA FAT-BURNING TECHNIQUES   145

9   COSMETIC SURGERY AND FAT   167

10   KEEP IT OFF! THIS MEANS THE FLAB!   181

BIBLIOGRAPHY   199

INDEX   201

ABOUT THE AUTHOR   207

APPENDIX   209

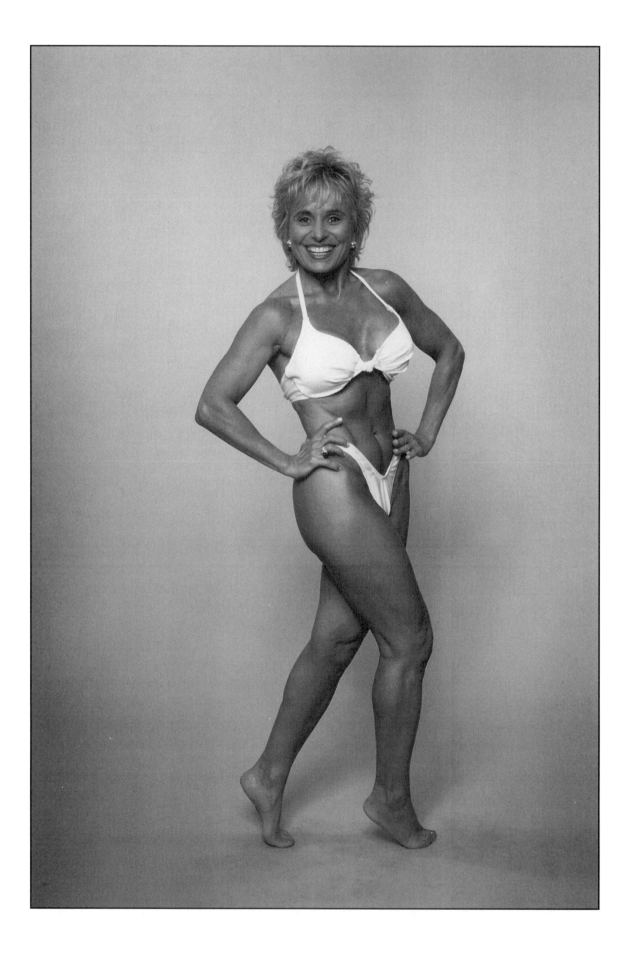

1

RECLAIM YOUR WAIST, HIPS, THIGHS, AND BUTT

Perhaps warmer weather is approaching, or maybe your planned vacation is coming up soon, but despite the promise of sunshine, you're filled with dread. It's bathing suit time! You picture yourself desperately searching through the stores to find a suit that will hide a multitude of sins. Well, there's good news.

You won't have to hide anything if you don't want to, and whether you choose to wear a conservative one-piece bathing suit or a daring bikini, you'll be proud of yourself and you'll never again have to dread donning a bathing suit. What's more, you'll be happy when you catch a glance of yourself when passing a mirror—in your underwear or even in the nude.

How long will this take? Here's the best part: *You can achieve a bathing suit body in thirty workout hours—and you can opt to put those hours in as fast as possible.* You can go on the 911 plan, where you zap your problem areas every day, or you can take the more relaxed road and work out every other day. You can do the regular plan, where you put in ten minutes a day, or the emergency plan, where you put in fifteen minutes a day. You can do it in record time because you'll be concentrating *only* on the problem areas, the spots that snug spandex does nothing to hide.

Busting the Bulge in Record Time

Most women have it—at least the women I've met, the women in the real world. It's that area in the middle of the body—you can even draw a circle around it. It begins at your waistline, goes down the front of your thighs to your knees, zooms around to your hips, butt, and back thighs. It's the area that inspires us to cover in the safety of a voluminous T-shirt, the area we are determined to hide, to cover up!

I have good news for you. Finally, once and for all, you can flatten your stomach and reclaim your waistline, firm and shape your thighs—both front and back—rid them of cellulite in the process, bomb away the bulges from your hips, and reduce the size of your butt, while at the same time shaping and lifting it. You can do it whether you're a "fat-fat" (significantly overweight—in which case you'll also follow the eating plan in Chapter 7) or a "skinny-fat" (not really overweight, but flabby or badly out of shape).

How do you do this? Follow this new exercise plan that will *zap* that "bathing suit area" in a rapid-fire sequence of exercises designed to get you fit and firm—fast!

The Secret of This Workout: The Zap-the-Fat "Tri-Set"

In this book you will find a workout method not found in any of my other books: the tri-set. Simply explained, a tri-set takes three complementary muscle groups and exercises them in sequence, without stopping. You will work your three most troublesome body parts one after another: hips/buttocks, thighs (both front and back), and your stomach (upper and lower—that "pooch"—and your waistline). You'll be zooming around the circle of fat without resting.

Only after you have done one full revolution will you rest for fifteen seconds. (Later, when you get used to the workout, you can even opt to eliminate that rest, burning more fat and reducing your exercise time in the process.) You will continue to use the fat-zapping tri-set until you've transformed your body into a firm, defined, shapely vision of feminine muscularity.

The Magic Seven—The Emergency Ten

There are seven mandatory revolutions in all, with three additional cycles for those of you who are in an emergency and want to get into bathing suit shape as fast as possible.

Never Be Bored! It's Over Before You Know It

The secret of the tri-set is, that it presents a relatively painless way of exercising. You never get bored, and you never get a chance to feel fatigued, because you are doing three completely different exercises in sequence, rather than the same old thing over and over again. In this workout, you will do one exercise for hips/buttocks, one exercise for thighs, and one exercise for the stomach without stopping. But even though you keep moving, certain body parts are resting and recuperating.

Here's how it works. While your hips/buttocks muscles are working, your thighs and stomach are resting, and while your thighs are working, your hips/buttocks and stomach are resting, and while your stomach is working, your hips/buttocks and thighs are resting. *But you don't rest.* You keep going, and going, just like a certain bunny we know, burning maximum fat and tightening, toning, and defining your bathing suit area.

Thirty Workout Hours to the Bathing Suit Body of Your Dreams

How long will it take you to get rid of your circle of fat and to replace it with lean, firm muscle? It all depends upon how quickly you put in those thirty workout hours. If you do the maximum plan, you'll get there faster than you will if you do the minimum plan, but in either case you'll get there. If you are overweight, you'll follow the bathing suit eating plan—and you'll watch your fat melt away and uncover a tight, toned, feminine body. You will either achieve your goal in thirty workout hours or show so much improvement that you won't give up the workout until you do! (Details on what to expect are found in Chapter 3, "Before and After.")

But They Say You Can't Get Rid of Cellulite

Sound of buzzer. Yes you can! You may have heard people say, "Cellulite is genetic." It is true that some people are more inclined toward "cottage cheese thighs" when they are overweight and/or out of shape, but the only reason for this is "thin skin." That's right. Most of us have bunched-up fat beneath the surface of the skin, but the thinner your skin, the more it shows. If you are among the thin-skinned, don't worry. By following this workout and following the bulge-busting diet, you will replace your cellulite with sleek muscle.

What exactly is cellulite anyway? Cellulite isn't a medical term. It's a term that was coined in the midseventies to describe bunched-up fat, fat that gives the appearance of an orange peel. This fat is made up of enlarged fat cells that conglomerate just beneath the surface of the skin, clinging to fibrous tissue for support.

As you follow my low-fat, balanced eating plan *and* you do the exercises in this workout, you build solid muscle under the skin, and eventually, the cellulite-ridden area smooths out. No more orange-peel. No more craters. Just curving contours of firm skin.

At first you may find one or two lingering dimples. But if you continue to do this workout, and to follow the eating plan, over time even those few remaining dimples will probably disappear.

No Equipment Necessary

What? Am I kidding? No equipment? That's right. Except for optional dumbbells (handheld weights) for the thigh exercises, you need absolutely nothing to do this workout—nothing except yourself. This means you can do this workout at home, in the office, on vacation—anywhere, anytime, anyplace.

If you want to invest in the optional dumbbells, all the better. You'll get a more intense thigh workout. And in time, as your thighs grow stronger, you have the option of trading in your five-pound dumbbells for tens, and eventually fifteens or even twenties. You may want to do this if you have the sagging thigh problem—you know, where the skin from your lower thigh drops over your knee—the result of Father Time! (A discussion on when to do this is found on p. 52.)

Ten Minutes a Day!

Once you get used to the routine, you will be able to breeze through it in just over ten minutes. How is this possible? It only takes ten to fifteen seconds to perform a set of exercises. You will be doing three sets of each of seven tri-sets, consisting of three exercises each, or twenty-one sets in total for the regular workout. Twenty-one sets of fifteen seconds each takes five minutes and fifteen seconds. But you are resting fifteen seconds between each tri-set. That means you will take six rests. So add a minute and a half for the rests. Now you have seven minutes and forty-five seconds. And six of the exercises are done on one side of the body at a time, so add fifteen seconds times six—another minute and a half—making the grand total ten minutes and fifteen seconds.

Bear in mind that you work more quickly once you get used to the workout. In addition, you can eventually eliminate all the rests. In time, you can finish the regular workout in seven minutes or less.

In the beginning, while you're learning to do the moves correctly and safely and while your body is getting used to the new challenge, the workout will take you longer—maybe as long as twenty to thirty minutes. But that won't last. You'll see. And anyway, unless you are a seasoned exerciser, you won't be doing the entire workout in the beginning. You'll be using a break-in-gently plan where you do no more than one third of the full workout. By the time you get to the full workout you'll be confident and up to speed!

Eleven to Fifteen Minutes for Quicker Results

For those of you who choose to add in one, two, or three exercises and do the Iron Woman, Steel Woman, or Titanium Woman workouts, add a minute or so each. The Iron Woman workout takes eleven minutes, the Steel Woman workout takes twelve minutes and forty-five seconds, and the Titanium Woman workout takes fourteen and a half minutes.

So there you have it. By investing only ten to fifteen minutes a day, and not even every day (you can work out three to six days a week—workout plans are discussed on pp. 43–44), you will have the bathing suit body of your dreams.

Why Isn't Dieting Enough to Get Your Hips/Buttocks, Thighs, and Stomach in Shape?

If you are overweight, dieting is absolutely necessary to get your middle body in shape. In fact, it is exactly this area of the body that provides the main storehouse for excess body fat. *But dieting alone cannot do the job.* No matter how strict your diet, once the fat is gone, unless you work out the right way, your body will feel soft and mushy and, even worse, your skin will sag. You may end up looking like a "skinny-fat."

The truth is, all you can hope to achieve from dieting alone is to fit into a smaller size. Dieting can't make your bathing suit area firm and shapely, nor can it give you definition. Only working out the right way can sculpt your body. You must do a series of specially designed exercises in a specific sequence in order to tighten, tone, and define your hips/buttocks, thighs, and abdominal muscles.

How We Get Tight and Toned

How does exercising the right way do the job? As you repeat a certain number of movements in a specific sequence, inevitably the muscle responds to the "work" being demanded of it. By moving the designated body part at carefully designed angles and planes, your working muscle eventually becomes not only stronger and harder (the muscle cells and fibers strengthen, become more concentrated, and increase, but it also begins to take on a new shape. In other words, your out-of-shape body part will become reshaped by the work being required of it; you will go from flabby to tight, toned, and defined. Your toned muscle is firm to the touch and pleasing to the eye. In addition, the body part becomes stronger—able to do more without becoming tired.

Don't worry that you will look like a bodybuilder if you do this workout. Bodybuilders use heavy weights and work out for hours every day to achieve an exaggerated muscularity. The only weights you will be using for this workout are optional light handheld weights for your thighs. If you wish to put on more muscle, you can go heavier—up to twenty pounds. Bear in mind, however, that female bodybuilders use heavy weights for thigh work—two hundred pounds, not twenty.

What about the rest of the body? This book concentrates on areas most critical to women, the bathing suit area. Later, if you want to shape up the rest of your body, you can get one of my total-body workouts or videos. I discuss this in detail in Chapter 10.

What about Aerobics?

Aerobic exercises are great for getting your heart and lungs into shape and for burning overall excess body fat. Also, being in "aerobic shape" makes all physical activity easier, including the workout in this book. If you are in aerobic shape, you won't get out of breath as quickly as you did before—and you may even be able to eliminate all the rests in this workout. But aerobics, with all their health benefits, won't transform your body. They won't make you look fabulous in a bathing suit. Only targeting specific muscle groups with certain exercises can do that.

Why do people think they can get their thighs in shape, for example, by using a stair-stepping machine? They believe that the repeated movement of the body part will reshape that body part. This movement does help to strengthen the thighs and hips/buttocks, but it cannot sculpt and define the thighs and lift the skin that sags over the thigh to the knee, or lift and shape the butt. Why? You're doing too many repetitions of one exercise without a rest, and you are not hitting the muscle from a variety of angles.

Bodybuilders whose entire careers depend upon body shaping realized this long ago. If aerobics could reshape the body, bodybuilders the world over would be hopping up and down, grapevining or jogging their way to definition. But the truth is that many bodybuilders don't even do aerobics, and those who do rely upon them only for heart and lung conditioning and extra fat burning. Body reshaping is a science. You have to do it a certain way, in a certain sequence, and from certain angles.

Should you forget about aerobics? Of course not. In fact, I advise you to do three to six twenty-to-forty-minute aerobic sessions a week. See Chapter 8 for more about this.

What Kind of a Diet Will Be Required?

Don't worry. I'm not going to ask you to starve to death. In fact, you'll eat plenty of food, and there will be a selection of foods that you can eat anytime, night or day, as much as you want. But you will have to reduce your fat intake and limit most foods. What's more, you will have to eat more often!

Anyone Can Do It—Create Your Own Workout!

There are thirty exercises in this workout, each targeting a specific area of your bathing suit area: waist and stomach, hips, butt, and front and back thighs. No matter how fat you are and regardless of your medical problems (you can work with your doctor), you can create a program tailor-made for you. In other words, you have a selection of so many exercises that even if you cannot (or will not) do certain exercises the Bathing Suit Workout contains enough options for you to create a plan that will work for you. More about this in Chapter 5.

What You Can Expect from This Workout

- A tight, toned stomach: upper stomach, lower "pooch," a trim waistline

- Higher, rounder, tighter buttocks and no saddlebags

- Firm, shapely front and back thighs

- Removal of cellulite

- Increased energy and self-confidence

- The lifetime fitness maintenance plan

- If overweight, reduced dress sizes—up to a size every three weeks

- If overweight, a delicious eat-till-you-drop (if you wish) fat-loss plan

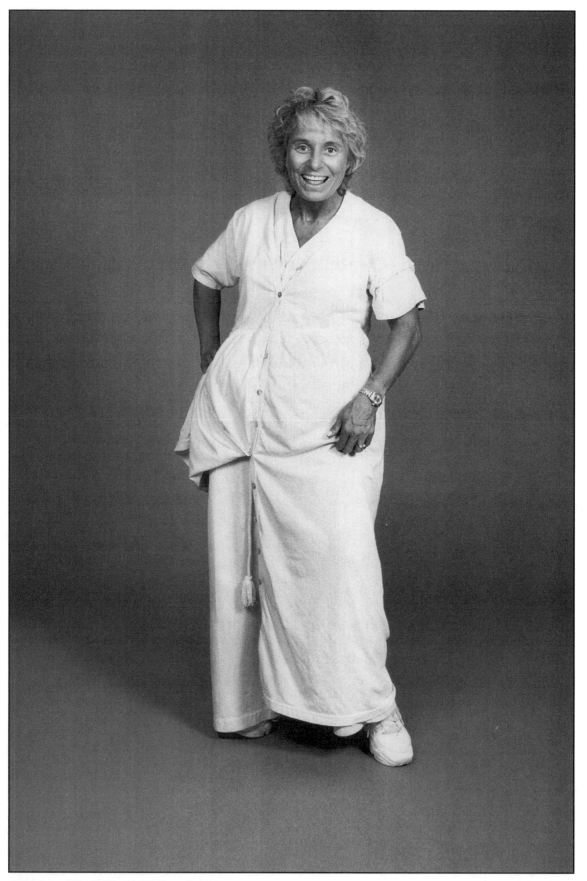

What I would look like if I didn't work out!

2

THE SKINNY
ON FAT!

You may have heard the expression "The rich get richer and the poor get poorer." For my purposes, I'd like to rephrase that. The rich get richer and the fat get fatter, and Americans, both rich and poor, are fat. Yes, despite the increased efforts of our health and fitness professionals and even the government itself, recent studies show that more Americans are overweight and out of shape than ever before. In fact, whereas only one fourth of adults were found to be overweight between 1960 and 1981, more than one third of adults are now considered overweight.

Why do people, in spite of all the emphasis on health and fitness, continue to grow fatter? Aside from the fact that we live in an increasingly sedentary society, in my opinion the answer is quite clear. People want to enjoy their lives, and they believe that eating what they want when they want is a big part of that enjoyment. Furthermore, they believe (wrongly) that in order to lose weight they would have to sacrifice eating pleasure forever.

If you are one of those people, I have some good news for you. You don't have to give up your eating pleasure completely, not even when you are losing your excess fat. Once you arrive at your fitness goal, you will be able to eat whatever you want once a week—and stay in shape for life. Because it contains the right combination of eating and exercise, the Bathing Suit Workout will show you a weight-loss plan you can stick to. In this chapter I'll talk about the food element that is the key to your weight-loss success—fat—and I'll explain why it tends to conglomerate on your stomach, hips, butt, and thighs. In Chapter 7, you'll get a full fat-loss diet!

To understand is to control. After reading this chapter, you will know the facts about fat—and this will help you to use your mind as a tool to control what you eat. Instead of resenting the fact that you must limit your fat intake as well as your overall daily calorie consumption, you will realize that it's the only logical thing to do, not only for your physical beauty, but for your health—indeed, for a longer, more energetic life.

What Is Contained in Food?

There are basic life-sustaining nutrients in all foods. These nutrients are broken down into three categories: water, micronutrients, and macronutrients. Water is the basic component of all foods. Without water we would die in a matter of days. Vitamins and minerals are the micronutrients found in all foods. They are needed in small quantities by the body. Without them we would suffer malnutrition and all kinds of unpleasant diseases. Carbohydrates, protein, and fats are macronutrients found in specific foods. They are required in greater quantities than any other food nutrients. However, for good health and a lean body, a careful macronutrient balance must be maintained. We should consume only about 12 to 15 percent of our total caloric intake in fat! (Most of the rest will be consumed in carbohydrates, and some in protein. I'll talk about this in Chapter 7.)

The Skinny on Fat

Fat is not all bad. In fact, it is absolutely necessary for the sustenance of your body, and indeed for your life. The problem with fat is not that we consume it, but that we consume too much of it. In fact, most Americans consume about 40 to 50 percent of their daily food intake in fat. The FDA says that for good health 30 percent of fat would be fine. Many medical doctors disagree. They feel that 20 percent would be a closer ideal percentage for good health, and even lower for fat loss. In fact, the Pritikin Longevity Center recommends that fat intake be as low as 10 percent, but never lower. Like most doctors, they agree that you will probably always feel hungry if your diet contains less than 10 percent fat. My fat-loss plan allows you to consume between 12 and 15 percent of fat—plenty to prevent hunger, and low enough to lose weight as fast as possible within the parameters of good health. You won't have to figure out percentages. I've done it for you by inventing a system where you only have to count fat grams. More about this later.

Why Do We Need Fat to Live?

It is fat that supplies the body with what are called "essential fatty acids." These are fatty acids that cannot be produced by the body itself, but must be supplied by fat intake from foods. These fatty acids are used by the body to produce hormonelike compounds that help to control blood clotting, blood pressure, and a host of other bodily operations. It is fat that comprises most of the cell membrane and sex hormones and helps to maintain healthy skin and hair. It also helps to transport fat-soluble vitamins D, A, E, and K through your bloodstream and helps to regulate your blood cholesterol level. You also need a certain amount of fat to cushion your internal organs. In addition, as mentioned above, if you keep your fat grams too low you will always feel hungry and you'll keep "picking" or "grazing." I used to do that until I wrote *Eat to Trim* (see Bibliography on p. 200) and upped my fat and lost twelve pounds—and I've kept those pounds off for over two years now. My new knowledge of fat and eating a balanced diet, in addition to the workout, is responsible for this success.

Why a Too-Low-Fat Diet Can Cause Overeating

If you don't have a certain amount of fat in your diet, no matter how much of other foods you eat, you'll still feel hungry because fat slows down the emptying of food from your stomach. You may find yourself constantly going back to the refrigerator. What you are really looking for is fat, but since you have forbidden yourself to eat it, you "pick," filling up on calorie-laden fat-free foods until you *gain* weight, even on a low-fat diet.

So don't become a fanatic and decide to eliminate all fat. If you consume 15 percent (about 15 to 25 grams of fat per day) of your total calorie intake in fat, you'll give yourself the benefit of the feeling full and at the same time you'll keep your fat intake low enough to lose as much weight as possible.

I'm not really worried that you will eliminate *all* fat from your diet. It would be very difficult to do so. There is at least a modest amount of fat in most foods. Even the humble apple has a gram of fat, and the lowest of low-fat protein fish and chicken sources have about one to two grams of fat per ounce. In Chapter 7 I'll give you a list of appropriate low-fat foods for your daily intake.

How We Get Fat

Simply put, we get fat when we eat more calories than we burn. As you may know, it takes 3,500 excess calories to cause one pound of fat to be stored on your body. But what are calories? A calories is a unit of chemical energy released to your body when you digest the food you have consumed. All foods contain calories, and you burn them all the time—when you're sleeping, and even breathing, burns about sixty calories an hour.

You Are What You Eat! Fat Calories Are Fatter than Other Calories

If you eat a high percentage of fat, you'll be fat! Why? There are more than double the number of calories in fat than in any other food. Fat has nine calories per gram while protein and carbohydrate have only four calories per gram. Obviously, it is much more diet efficient to eliminate as much fat from your food as you can than it is to go after protein and carbohydrate. (Later, I'll explain why carbohydrates are really the best food bargain of all.)

Fat gets even fatter! In fact, it is so fat and lazy that it does not go through the normal digestion process. When protein and carbohydrate are digested, they consume 20 to 25 percent of their own calories. But when fat is digested it uses up only 2 to 3 percent of its calories. It skips the whole cycle and goes straight to the place where it will be stored on your body—probably your hips, buttocks, thighs, and stomach.

Let's take a closer look at how this works. If you consume 100 calories of pure fat, say, for example, you eat a huge lump of full-fat cream cheese (standing at the refrigerator with spoon in hand—I've done it many times), after digesting that food, ninety-seven of those calories go straight to your fattest body part. In my case, it would be my stomach. But what if you ate a hundred calories' worth of nonfat pretzels instead? Only about seventy-five to eighty of those calories would be available for fat storage (20 to 25 percent has been burned up in the digestion process).

So you can see why if your goal is to lose your excess body fat, the only intelligent thing to do is to maintain a low daily intake of fat. Later you'll be able to indulge in any foods you wish once a week. But first you must reach your fitness goal. (I'll explain this in Chapter 7.)

Is It Percentage or Grams? How Do You Figure Out How Much Fat You Can Eat in a Day?

Good news here. Although I've been explaining fat consumption in terms of percentage, I rely on a system that allows you not to have to think about percentage. What do I have against percentage? Nothing, except that figuring percentage is too much work, and from the letters I get, I'm not the only one who feels this way. Most people I know forgot the small amount of math they learned in school. In fact, just thinking about figuring out percentages drives them to eat! With this in mind, I've simplified the whole thing for you by asking only that you do some addition.

In order to be sure that you're eating within the allowed 12 to 15 percent daily fat allowance, all you have to do is add up the fat grams you consume in a day and make sure that you don't go over twenty to twenty-five grams a day. On a bad day, I'll allow you to eat an extra five grams of fat, giving you a grand total of thirty grams. That would still keep you well within the fat-loss range.

Now that the FDA has required that all food labels list the fat grams per serving, your job of counting daily fat gram intake has been made delightfully easy. For the foods that come fresh, such as poultry or fish, you can refer to Chapter 7 or look them up in any fat gram counter (you can find a variety of them in any bookstore).

"98 Percent Fat Free" Can Be Misleading

When you see a food label that says "98% fat free" or some other seemingly impressive percentage, don't be fooled. The food may still contain a good deal more fat than is worth your expenditure.

Let me give you an example. I recently got a letter from a woman who sent me the label for Irish cream coffee. It said that the coffee was 98 percent fat free, but it had three fat grams per serving. She told me that she likes to have three or four cups a day. That would add up to nine to twelve grams of fat—half of her daily fat intake. Ridiculous! Why waste *any* fat grams on coffee, and who cares if it is 98 percent fat free? (And by the way, any regular or decaffeinated coffee without cream or sugar has zero fat grams.)

Is It Okay to Eat "Good Fat" (Polyunsaturated), the Kind That Does Not Clog Your Arteries?

No. Even though polyunsaturated fat is better for your health than saturated fat, it has the same amount of calories per gram as any fat, and will indeed make you just as fat.

For your information, saturated fats are found in animal products such as beef, pork, lamb, full-fat milk, cheese, and butter—and in addition, the vegetable products palm, palm kernel, and coconut oil. Except for the vegetable oils, all saturated fats become solid at room temperature. These fats cause elevated cholesterol levels, which in turn build up a solid material in your arteries, plaque, which in turn serves as a roadblock to your blood circulation. The result: heart attack.

And don't be fooled by "trans fatty acids," which are often billed as being good for your health. They can keep you just as chubby. These fatty acids are found in hydrogenated and partially hydrogenated oils contained in items such as potato chips, crackers, cookies, granola bars, and margarine. They tend to function in the body as saturated fats and can also clog your arteries.

Polyunsaturated fats (they come from vegetables, seeds, and nuts) are different. They are in liquid form and when consumed do not contribute to arteriosclerosis.

Is Cholesterol Fat?

No. Cholesterol is not fat, but a waxy, fatlike substance. It is found in nonfatty foods such as shrimp, eel, and squid and other seafood, and in fatty foods, such as red meats.

Like fat, cholesterol is not all bad. In fact, cholesterol is essential for life. Our cell membranes and nerve linings, brain, liver, and blood contain cholesterol, and cholesterol helps to form adrenal and sex hormones, bile, and vitamin D. It travels to body tissues in the bloodstream in lipoprotein—tiny droplets surrounded with a thin coating or shell-like material. These droplets transport cholesterol to and from body tissues. Cholesterol is naturally produced by your liver; you don't have to go out of your way to consume it.

Good Cholesterol, Bad Cholesterol

While we're on the subject of cholesterol, let's clear up the matter of "good" (HDL) and "bad" (LDL) cholesterol. Bad cholesterol tends to deposit itself on the arterial walls, forming the plaque that clogs arteries and prevents blood from flowing to the heart, causing heart problems that may lead to death.

Interestingly "good" cholesterol does the exact opposite of "bad" cholesterol. It helps to unclog the arteries by removing "bad" cholesterol from the bloodstream and transporting it out of the cells and into the bile and intestines, where it leaves the body through excretion.

But how do you know if you have too much of the wrong kind of cholesterol? You must take a fractionated cholesterol test. This test will give you what is called a cholesterol index. The lower your index, the lower your bad cholesterol and the lower your risk of heart attack. An index of four or lower is considered safe and healthy.

Just in case you're interested, an index is determined by dividing your total cholesterol by your good cholesterol (HDL). Let me give you an example. If your total cholesterol level is 200 and your HDL is 50, since 50 goes into 200 four times, your index is four.

Where's the Fat?

Okay. Now that you know what you know about fat, it's time to face up to the fact that until you get to your goal, certain foods are out of the question. They are:

All fried foods

Butter, margarine, lard, chicken fat, or oil (except very small amounts of olive or canola oil)

Mayonnaise with fat, and any fat-containing salad dressing

Peanut butter

Any ice cream, sour cream, cream cheese, and cheese that is not fat free

Milk, cottage cheese, or yogurt with more than 1 percent fat

Nuts, seeds, or any kind of "chips" (potato, corn, etc.)

Doughnuts, chocolate, croissants

Beef, bacon, lamb, or veal

Olives, avocados

Why such a long list? Anything on this list would be far too costly to your allowance of twenty to twenty-five grams of fat a day. You just can't afford them and stay within your budget. Let me give you some examples so you can see for yourself.

Food Product	Fat Grams
Fast-Food Hamburgers	
Burger King Whopper	36
Burger King Whopper with Cheese	45
Burger King Double Whopper	52
Burger King Double Whopper with Cheese	62
McDonald's Big Mac	36
Wendy's Single Plain Burger	15
Carls Jr. Country Fried Steak	33
Other Fast-Food Beef	
Arby's club sandwich	30
Arby's super roast beef sandwich	28
McDonald's Sausage McMuffin with egg	27.4
Arby's turkey sandwich	24
Burger King ham-and-cheese sandwich	24
Hot dog	15
Fast-Food Fried Chicken	
4-ounce thigh	19
4-ounce drumstick	16
4-ounce breast	15
Fast-Food Fish	
Arthur Treacher's fried fish	19.7
Arthur Treacher's fish sandwich	19.2
Croissant Foods	
Croissant	11
Burger King Croissan'wich with meat, egg, and cheese	24
Fast-Food Mexican Food	
Corn dog	16
Jack in the Box super taco	17
Taco Bell burrito	20
4 ounces refried beans with sausage	32
Fast-Food Potato Dishes	
Burger King french fries	22
Wendy's baked potato with cheese	24
Fast-Food Dessert Products	
Dairy Queen banana split	15
Large Dairy Queen ice cream dipped in chocolate	20

1 Ounce Cheese (One Slice)

Cheddar	9.4
American	8.9
Roquefort	8.7
Munster	8.5
Edam	7.9
Swiss	7.8
Limburger	7.7
Provolone	7.6
Mozzarella	6.1

You might be thinking that, compared to a Whopper hamburger, cheese doesn't seem so bad. But it is. It wouldn't be so terrible if you were willing to sacrifice the six to nine grams of fat for one slice of cheese as long as you kept within your daily twenty-five-fat-gram limit. The problem is, one slice of cheese never satisfied anyone I know. Eat one slice and the cheese starts calling you: "Just one more tiny morsel." Finally you give in and decide, "I'll just have a half." Then you promptly eat the whole slice, and then another, and then another. So forget about it. Stay away from cheese until you reach your goal. Then, once a week, you can have it.

What about low-fat cheeses? I think they are still too high in fat. The lowest of low-fat cheeses have one or two grams of fat per slice (ounce), and the highest nearly five grams per slice. What about nonfat cheese? Okay. But be careful. Calories count too if you overdo it. More about that in Chapter 7.

Ask Questions and Read Your Labels Carefully

Sometimes innocent foods such as granola, a cup of dried noodles (the kind you add water to), a salad, or even pasta can contain more fat than you ever imagined. For example, who would believe that Quaker 100% Natural granola cereal has ten grams of fat in a meager half-cup serving? Most oatmeals have no more than one or two grams of fat per serving. A one-serving container of cup-of-noodle type foods often contains up to twelve grams of fat, and sometimes more! A seemingly innocent chef's salad at Jack in the Box has nineteen grams of fat and, worse, a taco salad at Taco Bell has sixty-one grams of fat. A simple serving of what should be a very-low-fat dish, pasta, at Shoney's, will cost you a whopping sixteen grams of fat. Be a fat investigator. Ask before you eat. Fortunately, most of these fast-food establishments now serve wonderful low-fat alternatives.

What about Pizza?

Pizza that is not dripping in cheese but is heavier on the veggies is the least of all evils when it comes to fast or fatty foods. At least you're getting your nutrition's worth when you eat it—and in addition, it's filling. You won't feel as hungry after you eat a veggie pizza that's light on the cheese as you will with, say, two slices of cheese that contain even more fat.

If you are in an emergency and no other food is available, it's okay to eat a slice of pizza. One medium slice of my favorite pizza from Pizza Hut has ten grams of fat. You could get away with a slice if you watched your fat intake for the rest of the day and made sure you didn't go over your twenty-five grams. You could also blot the pizza with a napkin before eating to get rid of some of the melted fat.

What Do Sugar and Refined Carbohydrates Have to Do with Fat?

Sugar and refined carbohydrates, such as white bread, sourdough bread, fruit juices, sugar candy, jams and jellies, etc., can hinder the fat-burning process. How so? They cause the glucose to travel through your system so quickly that your insulin level rises. When this occurs, the enzyme (hormone-sensitive lipase) responsible for pulling fat from your cells is hindered. Fat is then trapped in your cells, and your body is forced to burn more carbohydrates and less fat. In addition, the rise in insulin stimulates your appetite. So keep your sugar and refined carbohydrates to a minimum (see p. 134).

Drinking Water Can Help Keep Fat off Your Body!

First and foremost, drinking plenty of water will help to calm down your appetite. It will also insure that you're not eating because your body is really dehydrated and craving the water in the food you will eat (foods are made up of at least 50 percent water).

In addition, water helps the body to metabolize its stored fat. Studies have revealed that when water intake is greatly decreased, fat deposits are increased. On the other hand, when water intake is increased, fat deposits are decreased. It works something like this: In order to function properly, the kidneys require a certain amount of water. When deprived of this water, they don't work to capacity, and the liver takes over their job. One of the main functions of the liver is to metabolize fat. However, since the liver is busy doing the work of the kidneys, it can't devote its full attention to metabolizing fat, and *it metabolizes less fat*. This fat remains stored in the body. I now drink at least eight eight-ounce glasses of water a day.

Where Is Your Main Fat Storage Bin?

For women, the major part of fat is stored in the hips/buttocks, thighs, and abdominals (stomach). But which specific area of your body stores the most fat? Each woman is different. You can determine where you store the majority of your fat by looking in the mirror. Which body part *looks* the fattest? Is it your hips/buttocks area, your thighs, or your stomach? Another way to test where your first storage place for fat is to be aware of where the excess pounds show up first when you start to gain weight. Even when you are in near-perfect shape, it is this area that will hold on to those last few pounds of fat. I get letters from women all the time: "Your workout is great. But I still have one problem. My lower stomach . . ."

In order to get rid of that last bit of fat, you will have to keep your weight-loss eating plan very strict and bomb away at that body part with extra exercises. You'll be doing both if you follow this book exactly as written.

Body Fat Percentage

Some women have a body fat percentage as high as 65 percent. The average American woman has about half that amount, 33 percent Medical authorities seem to agree that a fit woman should have a body fat percentage of about 22 to 23 percent. Interestingly, my body fat is about 22 percent—not as low as you would think! Do I care? Not at all. The only reason I had my body fat measured in the first place was to answer the question so my fans who said, "I'll bet your body fat percentage is about ten percent." For me, that will never happen. Part of it is genetic, and part of it is that I love to eat.

The way I see it, I look good enough the way I am. I want to enjoy my life, and eating happens to be one of the things I enjoy. At my age, I'm not planning on winning a beauty contest or becoming a model, and there's no reason for me to be bone thin. (Anyway, I don't think I would have won such a prize at any age, or have been qualified as a model—I'm too short, not to mention other things.) If you take a close look at my photos, you will notice that I do carry some excess body fat on my stomach and hips/buttocks. I do care, but not enough to give up eating altogether! I love food.

What Is Brown Fat?

You may have heard of something called brown fat, as opposed to regular or yellow fat. It is found in blood vessels that lead to the heart, near the spine, and in the chest, in grapelike clusters. In the 1980s there was a great interest in this type of fat because it was discovered that such fat behaves like fat-burning furnace. In other words, people who have a proper supply of brown fat can get away with an occasional binge without the consequence of weight gain.

I can just imagine what you're thinking: "Tell me, tell me, how can I get this brown fat?" Until now, we don't know exactly how people get it, but we do know who has it, and those are the people who seem to need it the least: athletes who are already in shape. So why am I telling you this? If you follow this workout and get yourself in shape, and better yet, if you do the optional aerobics and follow through with a weight-training program for the rest of your body, you are likely to have more brown fat.

If brown fat really does what it is reputed to do, I think we should change its name to something other than fat. Why? To get fat, all you have to do is eat fat. But to get brown fat, you can't eat fat. In fact, you have to do something quite different. You have to work out and eventually be in the condition of an athlete.

Two Women: Same Height, Weight, Bone Structure—Yet One Looks So Much Fatter!

Just the other day I approached a woman in the gym who seemed to be my height and bone structure. She had just stepped off the scale, and I noticed that it said 116 pounds. As she gathered her gym bag, I weighed myself. I also weighed 116 pounds. But she looked much fatter than I did. On the way out of the gym, I asked her to guess my weight. "A hundred and five pounds," she said. "Nope. I'm a hundred and sixteen," I replied. She was amazed. I asked her what size dress she wears and she said, "Nine." I wear a three to five!

What followed was a discussion like the one in the following paragraphs. Muscle weighs more than fat but takes up less space. I have more muscle on my body than she does, and her feathery or spongelike lightweight fat is wider and bigger than my heavyweight, lean, dense muscle.

Do I make my point? Forget the scale and look in the mirror. As you put muscle on your body you'll see greater changes in the mirror than you will on the scale. You may lose five pounds of fat, but you may also be increasing muscle, so the scale may show little or no drop. But in the meantime you look and feel much leaner (I mean your body will literally feel harder). Please. I beg you. Let the scale be just a curiosity. Don't use it as a gauge to measure whether or not you are getting in shape. Let the mirror and the way your body feels be your guides.

How Can You Implant within Yourself a Fat-Burning Furnace that Operates Twenty-four Hours a Day?

Muscle is a permanent fat-burning furnace. How so? Muscle raises your basal metabolism—the minimum quantity of energy you use even when resting in order to sustain your life.

When you develop muscles on your body, you will use more energy (use up more calories and burn more excess fat) than you used to while doing the same activities. For example, if you used to burn sixty calories an hour sleeping, you will now burn about 20 percent more, say, seventy-two calories per hour. The more muscle you put on your body, the more you raise your basal metabolism, and the more fat you burn twenty-four hours a day. Champion bodybuilders burn at least twice as much or more fat twenty-four hours a day than average people—and in fact must eat twice as much or more than ordinary people in order to sustain their bodies. You can see why, if you love to eat, having muscles is a good idea!

How Can You Convince Your Discouraged Self that Once and for All You Can Get Rid of the Excess Body Fat?

You can get with the program. You can stop berating yourself for past failures and begin today. You can, by an act of will after reading this book, take the first step by placing the book on the floor, opening to the first exercises, and then "just doing it." That's right. One stroke at a time. One day a time. That's all it takes to begin a new life. And if you need extra encouragement, read my book *Look In, Look Up, Look Out: Be the Person You Were Meant to Be* (see Bibliography)—especially the chapter called "Motivate Yourself: Your Personal Bag of Tricks." That'll get you going for sure.

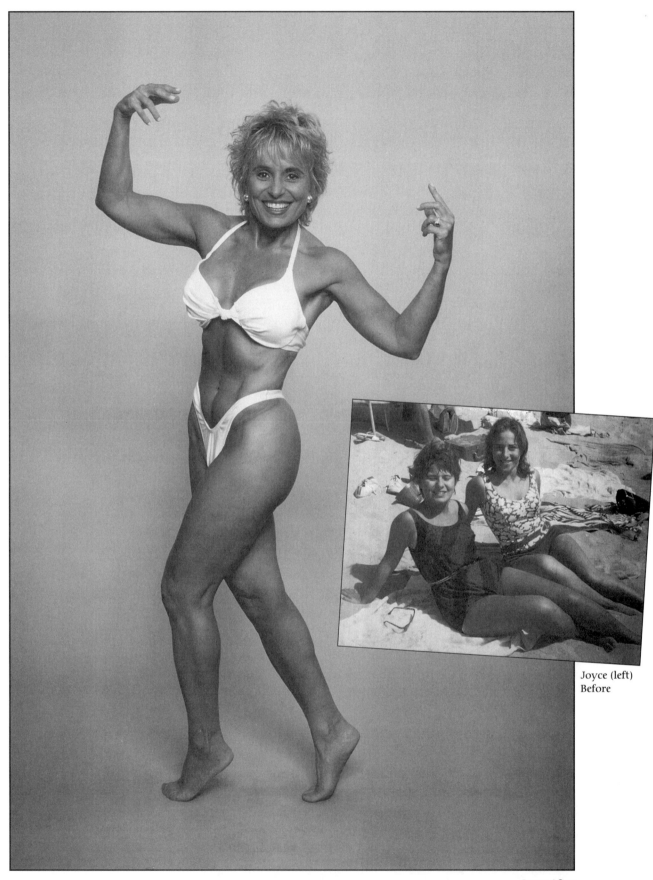

Joyce (left)
Before

Joyce After

3
BEFORE AND AFTER

Before and after! We all want results. That's what it's all about. The bottom line is, What can I expect to see as a result of this workout? In this chapter you will meet five women who did the Bathing Suit Workout and achieved a wonderful result. But first let's take a look at my before-and-after photos.

I finally dug up an old "fat" photo of myself when I was nineteen years old. I had gone from a "skinny" ninety-eight pounds to a fat 131—and then I stopped weighing myself. After that I went on many diets and, as discussed in my other books, I yo-yoed up and down over the years—but even when I lost the weight I was a "skinny-fat." It was only after learning the secrets contained in this (and other books I've written) that I was able to get in shape.

I've been doing the Bathing Suit Workout for my hip-butt-thigh and stomach area for the past year now and—Wow! I've never had a better "bathing suit body" in my life! In fact, I'm showing you my butt in a "thong" for the first time ever—and you are looking at a fifty-five-year-old butt! I would never do this before (show you a photo of myself in a thong), but I'll make the supreme sacrifice to make the point. (See p. 41 rear-anatomy shot for the photo of me in the thong.)

Now let's talk about the other "before-and-after" women.

Ivonne: Size 20 Before—Size 7 after Thirty Workout Hours

Look at Ivonne. She did the regular Bathing Suit Workout six days a week—and look at the results after thirty workout hours. It took her about twenty-six weeks. She did my Bottoms Up! Workout and, later, used *Definition* for the rest of her body.

"The first time I picked up your book, I hated your guts. What guts! Look at the body that that hussy has! *Wham!* Across the room you went. But finally—I went through many stages, it's a long story—I got started, and the rest is history.

"This past summer I vacationed in Cancún for two weeks. They were the happiest weeks of my life. Why? Because when I was younger, I was given nicknames such as Bon-Bon, which meant marshmallow. My brothers could not get enough of calling me Fatso. I missed out on a great deal, like proms, dates, and parties because of my weight. But thanks to you, now, at thirty-four, I look and feel my best, and I'm no longer ashamed of my body. I am now realizing my dreams—not just in looking good but in achieving goals and fulfilling my potential. I love you, Joyce Vedral—you're a very real person."

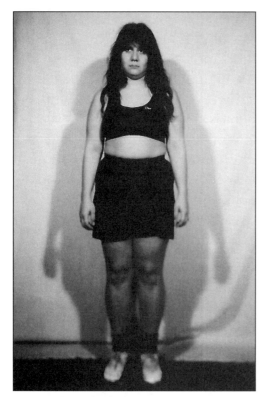
Ivonne Before, Size 20

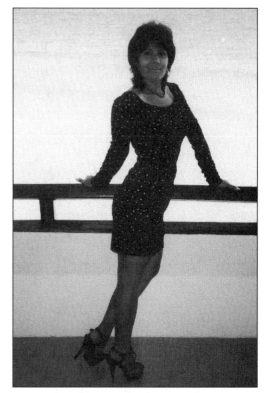
Ivonne after Thirty Workout Hours, Size 7

Chris: Size 16 Before—Size 8 after Thirty Workout Hours

Chris did the regular Bathing Suit Workout—ten minutes a day, four days a week—for forty-five weeks (thirty Bathing Suit Workout hours in all), and look at her now! She did the Fat-Burning Workout for the rest of her body.

"I've never felt so good in my life," says Chris. "It was fun buying

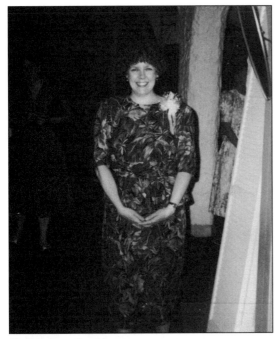

Chris Before, Size 16

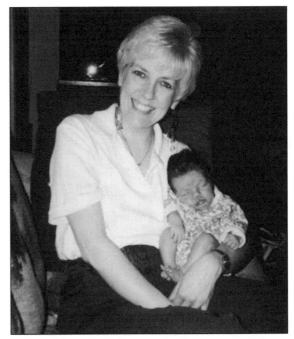

Chris after Thirty Workout Hours, Size 8

new clothes, going down the size rack—first a 16, then a 14—all the way down to size 8! I can't begin to tell you how many people I have told about this workout. Most of them don't believe me until I show them a 'before' picture. I get compliments all the time. I am constantly showing my muscles to people. So many people began doing what I'm doing—one girl at work lost over forty pounds. Thank you much, Joyce."

If Chris, who is forty-two years old, has two children, twelve and nine, and works full time as a legal secretary (she is a single mom), can do it, so can you. "I'm really busy, but I always find time to work out because I want to look good. I know that I'm old enough that if I let my body go and I don't start taking care of it, I'm going to be in big trouble. Also, I feel much better when I work out—as if I've accomplished something."

Anita: Size 13 Before—Size 9 after Thirty Workout Hours

Anita did the regular Bathing Suit Workout six days a week for thirty weeks and my Definition Workout for the rest of her body, and look at her now!

"I'm so pleased with the way I look. I never looked like this, even when I was a teenager. Every one I know, including the members of my family, agree. I get compliments all the time. I feel and look—well, people tell me I look—thirty-two, but I'm forty-five years old."

Anita told me that her whole life has changed for the better now that she doesn't have to worry about her body.

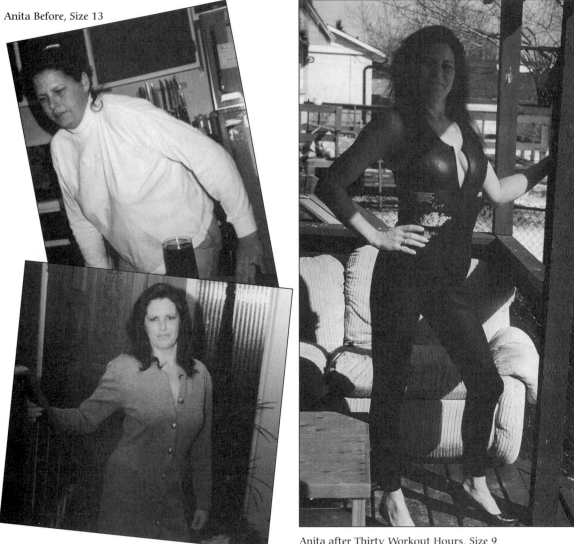

Anita Before, Size 13

Anita after Thirty Workout Hours, Size 9

Michelle: Size 12 Before—Size 9 after Twelve Workout Hours

Michelle first wrote to me when she had gone down from a size 22 to 24 to a size 14 in twenty-six weeks after using my book *The Fat Burning Workout*. She later switched to my books *Bottoms Up!* and *Definition*, and got down to a size 12 after another twelve weeks. That's how you see her in the before photo, a size 12.

I told Michelle that she looked fine the way she was, but she said,

"What about my middle? I feel I still need some special work there." So I sent her the manuscript to a new book I was working on—this book, *The Bathing Suit Workout*—and look what she did in twelve workout hours!

Michelle did the Titanium Woman workout from this book, fifteen minutes a day, three days a week. It took her sixteen weeks! She continues to switch back and forth between my other workouts for the rest of her body, among them Definition, the Fat-Burning Workout, and Bottoms Up! and the 12-Minute Total-Body Workout.

Michelle is thirty years old and has a four-year-old son. She also works as a data processor, so she is very busy and does not have a lot of time to work out. "I did my workout at my lunch hour with my friend. I've got a whole lot of people doing your workout now.

"In spite of my hectic schedule, I always find time to do it. At first it seemed like a lot of work, but in a week you get familiar with the exercises and you don't have to read how to do them anymore—and I love the tear-out wall charts.

"I can see my middle body, my stomach and my hip-butt-thigh area. They are a lot tighter and the jigglyness is completely gone."

Michelle Before, Size 12

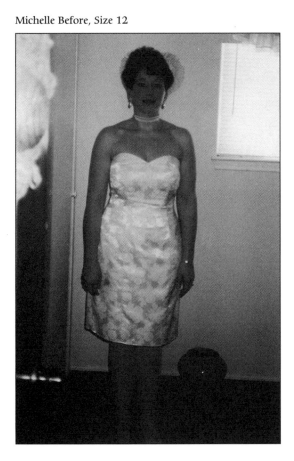

Michelle after Twelve Workout Hours, Size 9

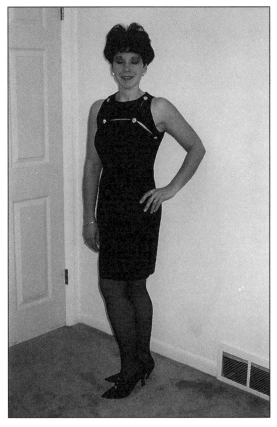

Kelley: Size 8 Before—Size 6 after Six Workout Hours

Kelley is thrilled with her results. She used my Fat-Burning Workout to get down from a size 16 to a size 8 in twelve weeks (sixteen workout hours). Then she used *The Bathing Suit Workout*, doing the maximum plan: the Titanium Woman workout three days a week for eight weeks (six workout hours), and look at her now!

Kelley says, "I'm a landscaper. I'm used to lifting fifty-pound bags—and you see how I looked in my before photo. So what was wrong with this picture? Why wasn't I in shape? Well guess what: It's not how much you're lifting or working, it's how you're working. Once I learned what to do, I got results so fast people don't believe me. And if you think I have time to spend hours working out, forget it. I'm thirty-six and I have three children—ten, thirteen, and fourteen! I get my workout done and out of the way. I used to go to a health club but I dropped it. It wasn't working. I can do this with so little effort. Not only do I look better, but I feel so much better too—stronger, more energy."

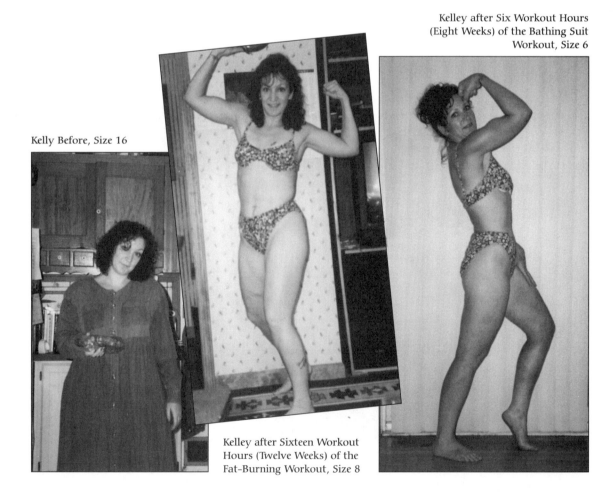

Kelley after Six Workout Hours (Eight Weeks) of the Bathing Suit Workout, Size 6

Kelly Before, Size 16

Kelley after Sixteen Workout Hours (Twelve Weeks) of the Fat-Burning Workout, Size 8

Small wonder. The stomach or midsection, as you may know, is the center of strength. I asked Kelley what she's doing now in the way of a workout. She said, "I devised my own plan—switching back and forth using all of your books in cycles of six weeks for the rest of my body. I'll use *The Fat Burning Workout* for six weeks, then switch to *Definition* for six weeks, then use *Bottoms Up!* or *Now or Never*. I even use (and love) *Top Shape* and *Gut Busters* for six weeks, and so on. I do this to challenge my muscles—so they won't get bored." Kelley tells me that she has all of her friends working out!

What About You?

Now that you've read the inspirational stories of other women, what about you? If it can happen to me and if it can happen to them, it can happen to you. You are not the exception to the rule. That is a lie you tell yourself because of your past false starts. This is not a false start. Begin today by taking a before photo of yourself and pasting it in the space below. Then finish reading this book, underlining text and making comments in the margins (this is the best way to really absorb the book). Then set a start date and go! Begin a workout that will change your life for the better in every way, shape, and form—not just physically but psychologically as well.

Your Before Photo   Your Photo after Thirty Workout Hours

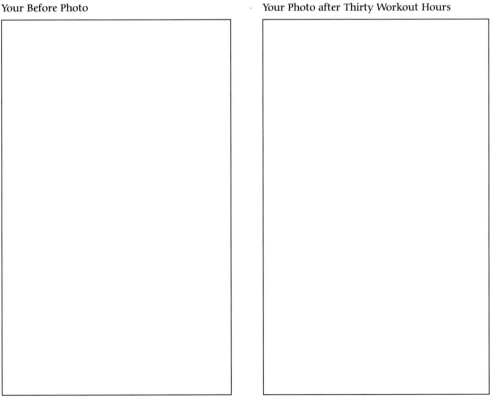

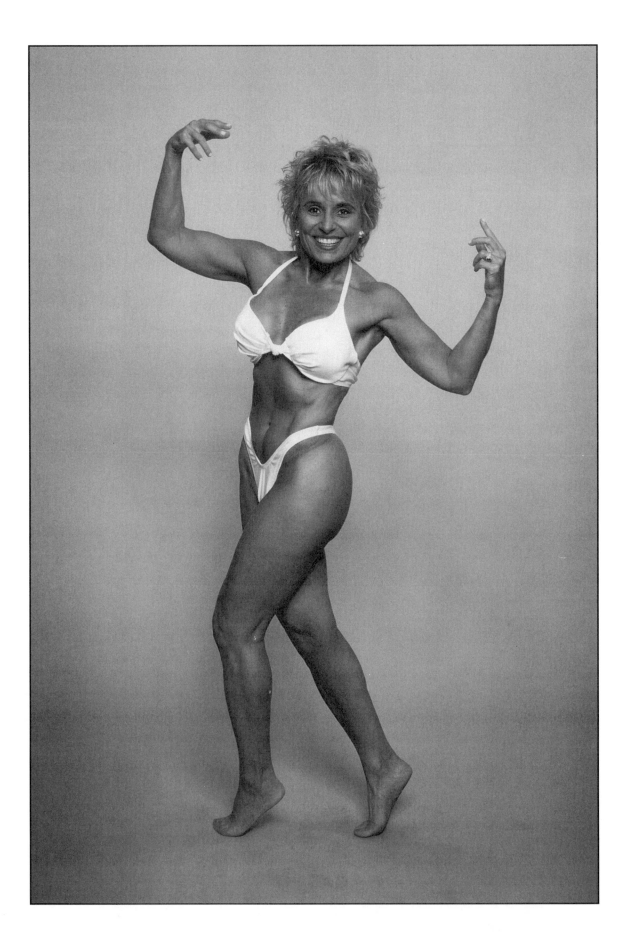

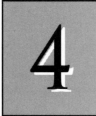

WHAT YOU NEED TO KNOW, WHAT YOU NEED TO FORGET!

In order to succeed at any workout, there are certain basic things you must know before you start. In addition to what you must learn, there are things you must forget! There are certain preconceived ideas based upon misinformation and preconditioning that must be removed from your thinking before you start the workout, so that your progress will not be hindered.

In the following paragraphs you will find basic operating information, which will help you to "clear the slate" of your mind so that you can start fresh and begin a workout that will, once and for all, end the problem you've had all of your adult life. No longer will your hips, buttocks, thighs, and stomach represent a vicious circle of frustration for you.

Exercise Information

An **exercise** is a specified movement for a given muscle, designed to encourage that muscle to become stronger, harder, shapelier, and more defined. For example, the knee-raised oblique crunch is an exercise designed to tighten, tone, and define the upper abdominal area.

A **repetition**, or rep, is one complete movement of an exercise, from start, to midpoint, to endpoint (which is really back to start). For example, one repetition of the saddlebag stripper involves lying on your side and raising your leg as high as possible (midpoint) and lowering your leg back to the original position (endpoint).

A **set** is a given number of repetitions of a specific exercise that are performed without a rest. In this workout one set will consist of fifteen repetitions. This will apply to all exercises in the workout.

A **superset** is the performance of two exercises without taking a rest. You can superset within body parts by doing two exercises for the same body part before you take a rest, or you can superset between body parts by doing two exercises for two different body parts before taking a rest. The superset is not used in this workout, but you will need to understand the term when thinking about the workouts described in Chapter 10.

A **speed superset** is a combined set of two exercises for the same body part, without taking a rest between supersets. In other words, you do all three sets for two exercises before you take a rest. The speed superset is not used in this workout, but you will need to know this term in order to understand the workouts described in Chapter 10.

The **speed set** is combined set of all sets of a given exercise, where the exercise stops only long enough to pick up the next weight. For example, if you were to choose to do your chest routine with speed sets rather than combining the flat bench press and the flat bench flye, you would perform all five sets of your flat bench press without resting. Then you would take a short rest and perform all five sets of your flat bench flye. The speed set is not used in this workout, but you will need to know the term in order to understand the workouts described in Chapter 10.

A **giant set** is a combination of three compatible exercises for the same body part without taking a rest. The giant set is not used in this routine, but you will need to know the term in order to understand other workouts, discussed in Chapter 10.

A **tri-set** is a combination of three compatible exercises for different body parts that are done without taking a rest. This entire workout will be based upon tri-sets of hips/buttocks, thigh, and abdominal exercises. Only after one set of exercises has been performed for each of those three body parts can a fifteen-second rest be taken.

The **speed tri-set** is the performance of one tri-set after another without taking advantage of the allowed fifteen-second rest. The advantage of this method is twofold: (1) you save time, and (2) you burn more fat. Note: It is only after you have become very adept at the workout that you can use the speed tri-set.

The **true or "regular" pyramid system** is the adding of weight to each set with a simultaneous reduction of repetitions until a peak is achieved, and then the reduction of weight on each set with a simultaneous addition of repetitions until the starting amount of weight and repetitions is once again achieved.

For example, in this workout, beginning exercisers would use the following pyramid:

Set 1: Twelve repetitions at one pound

Set 2: Ten repetitions at two pounds

Set 3: Eight repetitions at three pounds

Set 4: Ten repetitions at two pounds

Set 5: Twelve repetitions at one pound

The **modified pyramid system** is the adding of weight to each set at the expense of a few repetitions only until the peak of the pyramid is reached. For example:

Set 1: Twelve repetitions at one pound

Set 2: Ten repetitions at two pounds

Set 3: Eight repetitions at three pounds

Since for the most part no weights are used with this workout, neither the modified or true pyramid system is required. You can opt to use the modified pyramid system with your thigh routine. For absolute maximum results, I recommend that you use weights and the modified pyramid system for thighs. You will also need to be familiar with these terms in order to understand the information regarding other workouts in Chapter 10.

A **rest** is a pause between sets or exercises. The function of a rest is to allow the working muscle time to recover so that it can cope with the next set of exercise. As mentioned above, in this workout you will take a fifteen-second rest only after you have performed three exercises—one each for hips/buttocks, thighs, and abdominals. Your muscles can cope very well without resting for three sets because you are not exercising the same body part for three sets in a row. Indeed, you are exercising three different body parts. While one body part is working, the others are resting. But since you are still on the move, you continue to burn fat.

Breathing naturally while you exercise means to inhale and exhale unconsciously in an instinctive, as opposed to a thoughtful, manner and not to hold your breath. When performing a new or challenging exercise, many people tend to hold their breath. It's an unnecessary "survival instinct" tactic. You will notice that from time to time in the exercise instructions, I remind you to not hold your breath and ask you to breathe naturally.

Some experts believe that you should breathe out (exhale) on the flex part of the exercise, and breathe (inhale) in on the stretch part of the exercise. This would be necessary if you were lifting heavy weights, such as powerlifters do. For our purposes, it's better not to think about your breath at all. Focus all of your attention on your working muscles.

A **routine** is the specific combination of exercises prescribed for a certain body part. For example, in this workout your regular hips/buttocks routine consists of seven exercises: the saddlebag stripper, the lower butt curl, the lower butt crunch, the lower butt side kick, the floor feather kick-up, the lying butt lift, and the one-leg prone butt lift. The Iron Woman workout adds the standing butt squeeze. The Steel Woman workout adds the reverse-lunge lift, and the Titanium Woman workout adds the straight-leg kick-up. In this workout you will perform your abdominal routine in combination with your thighs and abdominals.

A **workout** includes all the exercises to be performed by the exerciser on a given day. For example, in this workout, you will perform seven tri-sets consisting of a hips/buttocks, thigh, and abdominal exercise for the regular workout, eight tri-sets for the Iron Woman workout, nine tri-sets for the Steel Woman workout, and ten tri-sets for the Titanium Woman workout.

The term **weight** refers to resistance, or the heaviness of the dumbbell used in a given exercise. In this workout, except for rare occasions, no weight is used for hips/buttocks or abdominal exercises, and graduated dumbbells can be used for all thigh exercises. (You will raise your weights as you get stronger.)

A muscle is **flexed** when the muscle fibers are shortened as the muscle is squeezed together. For example, your quadriceps (front thigh muscle) is flexed when you return to the start position from a regular squatting position. In this workout, I ask you to add to that natural flex by willfully squeezing your muscle as it flexes, adding to the force of the flex. You can help yourself to flex a muscle by imagining that someone is about to punch you hard in that muscle. Your natural reaction will be to contract or flex that muscle in defense.

A muscle is **stretched** when the muscle fibers are elongated. For example, your quadriceps (front thigh muscle) is stretched when you lower yourself to the squatting position. In the exercise instructions, I ask you to "feel the stretch" in various muscles.

Muscle isolation is the method of exercising each muscle completely and independently of other body parts. Muscle isolation is necessary in order to insure maximum muscle growth, development, and definition. Although this workout combines three exercises, the principle of muscle isolation is not violated because you are not working muscles at random. You are asked to perform three exercises in rapid sequence, and to return quickly to the previous muscle groups and repeat the cycle. The rest time between the exercising of your specific muscles is not long enough to hinder progress. On the other hand, if you skipped around at random, working various muscles on your body at will and taking your time, your muscles would rest too long and would not respond effectively to the challenge of the exercises.

Progression refers to the periodic adding of weight to specific exercises when the weight being used is no longer enough of a challenge. For example, in about four weeks you may feel that you are ready to use ten-pound dumbbells for your thigh exercises. Two months after that, you may see that you can use fifteen-pound dumbbells, and in another six months you may be able to advance to twenty pounds. But where does it end? Will you eventually be lifting fifty-, seventy-five-, and one-hundred-pound dumbells? Of course not. You will eventually reach a "plateau" where you will say to yourself, "I like what I see. I don't want to get bigger muscles." At this point you will keep the same weights forever.

Target date is the date you set for your visualized body to arrive! The date must be realistic. Then mark that date on the calendar and continually picture your body evolving into its ideal form by your target date.

A **plateau** refers to a weight ceiling where the exerciser can either remain or attempt to break through. Most people reach their weight-training plateau in about a year. At that time you may choose to remain at that plateau or go higher.

Technique Information: Altering the Effect of Your Exercises

An exercise routine becomes **aerobic** when it causes your pulse to reach 60 to 80 percent of its capacity, and to stay that way for a certain length of time. (Some authorities insist that in order to achieve an "aerobic effect," one must work for twenty minutes uninterrupted. However, more and more exercise specialists are beginning to agree that one achieves an aerobic effect in as short a time as ten minutes.)

You can figure out your maximum pulse rate by subtracting your age from 220 and then multiplying the result by 80 percent. You can find your minimum aerobic pulse by multiplying that number by 60 percent. If you follow this workout exactly as prescribed, taking the minimum number of rests, you will be well within the aerobic range. You don't have to check your pulse continually. If you break into a sweat after about seven minutes, rest assured that you are in the aerobic range. This workout is aerobic if you do not take advantage of the fifteen-second rest after each tri-set. But even if you do choose to rest the fifteen seconds, you get a significant fat-burning effect.

Intensity is the degree of difficulty or challenge of the exercise program you are following. Intensity can be increased by adding to the number of repetitions, increasing the load of weight, reducing the rest periods allowed between sets and between exercises, or using continual pressure. This is a very high-intensity workout because you are asked to do three exercises of fifteen repetitions each before you are allowed to take a rest. If you wish, you could increase the repetitions from fifteen to twenty-five, but frankly, the workout is already intense enough. I do only fifteen repetitions each.

Dynamic tension is the willful force exerted on a muscle as it is being stretched or elongated. In a normal situation when a muscle elongates, no pressure is exerted on the muscle. However, one can deliberately and consciously exert pressure on the muscle even as it elongates.

Isometric pressure is the willful force exerted on a muscle as it is being flexed or shortened, above and beyond the normal force used when flexing a muscle.

Continual pressure involves willfully squeezing (flexing) the muscle as hard as possible on the contraction part of the movement, and continuing to keep pressure on the muscle by deliberately using as much dynamic tension on the muscle as possible on the stretch part of the movement. Continual pressure is a combination of dynamic tension and isometric pressure. You will try to use continual pressure as much as possible as you do the Bathing Suit Workout.

Concentration is mentally focusing on the specific muscle you are exercising by watching, touching, and/or thinking about that muscle as you perform your repetitions, and by picturing that muscle becoming firm, strong, shaped, and defined. Concentration also involves actively "telling" the muscle to grow and be reshaped. (This helps the unconscious mind to go into action.)

Visualization is the picturing in your mind of what you want to have happen to your body. As you are working out, imagine the body part you are working being reshaped into the form you have in mind.

The **unconscious mind** can be used to help you to reach your fitness goal. Your conscious mind (you) "tells" your unconscious mind to get you to your goal in a certain, reasonable amount of time. For example, you've read this book and you're determined to get in shape. In order to employ your unconscious mind's help, stand in the mirror and "tell" your body to become reshaped by a certain reasonable date, and picture your body evolving into that shape. Your unconscious mind will begin to cooperate and alert you when you are tempted to skip a workout, do a lazy workout, or overeat. I often compare the unconscious mind to a homing torpedo or a Scud missile that zigzags its way toward its target once programmed because that's just what it does. It gets you to your goal on the target date, sometimes seemingly miraculously.

Details Concerning Muscles

Muscle mass is the specific size of a given muscle. In order to experience muscle growth, you must consistently challenge the muscle. Muscle mass is developed, shaped, and sculpted by the particular work or exercise it is being asked to do. For example, your front thigh muscles will become firm as a muscle is formed under the skin, replacing the fat (you will lose this as you follow the low-fat eating plan). Your front thigh muscles will also be sculpted into an appealing form and defined so as to look athletic and sexy.

Muscularity is a comparative term. It depicts the quantity of muscle on your body as opposed to fat. As you continue to do the Bathing Suit Workout and to follow the low-fat eating plan, your muscle-to-fat ratio will increase—that is to say, you will have a higher and higher percentage of muscle and a lower percentage of fat on your hips/buttocks, thighs, and abdominals.

Definition is the clearly delineated lines that separate muscles from each other and divide muscles themselves, and make them appear sculpted and separated. Well-placed definition can also help to give the body a more balanced, symmetrical look. For example, definition in the obliques (side abdominal muscles) draws attention away from a large waistline and causes the waist to appear smaller. The diagonal lines cause the waist to appear to slant in and look less boxy. My waist is twenty-seven inches—that's my bone structure. No matter how thin I get, my waist will never be smaller. Yet because of my definition in that area, most people think my waist is much smaller.

When one has extreme definition, one is considered to be **ripped**. After doing this routine for about six months, assuming that you have lost your excess body fat by following the low-fat eating plan, your abdominal muscles will appear to be ripped. They may in fact have what is called the beer-can look, so called for the six-pack of muscles inscribed on the stomach. (Quite the opposite of the beer-belly look.)

Density is the hardness of a muscle. A muscle is most dense when it has little intramuscular fat. The Bathing Suit Workout will eventually force the fat not only from under your skin where most of it resides, but from the muscle itself. When muscle density increases, muscles feel more firm to the touch.

Total body **symmetry** refers to the balance and proportion of all the muscles on your body in relation to all the other muscles on your body. In order to achieve total body symmetry, you will want to choose one of my full workout books and do exercises for the other six body parts: chest, shoulders, biceps, triceps, back, and calves. See Chapter 10 and the Bibliography for information on this.

The **forty-eight-hour recovery principle** is the allowing of forty-eight hours (or a day of rest) before rechallenging a muscle with a weight-training workout in order to allow the muscle optimum growth and to prevent overtraining and muscle attrition (wearing down). Traditionally, the only muscle that is an exception to this rule has been the abdominal area, because it is not exercised with weights. However, the buttocks are also not exercised with weights and can also be exercised day after day. In this workout, we will bend the rules and allow you to exercise your thighs consecutively because you will be using very light weights for your thighs. Later, when you get close to your size goal and you have increased the weights for your thigh exercises, you should do your Bathing Suit Workout every other day.

Split-routine is the exercising of a given number of body parts on workout day one, resting, or working on a different given number of body parts on workout day two, and so on.

The purpose and the necessity of the split routine is to allow the exercised muscle forty-eight hours' recovery time before it is challenged again. If you are using significant weights and do not allow this amount of rest time, a muscle may become exhausted from overtraining, and development will be slowed down or even reversed.

Sticking points are periods of time when, although you are working out regularly, no apparent improvement is visible. At such times progress *is* being made, only it is under the surface. Think of it as a seed in the ground. You don't know that anything is happening until the green bud pops through the earth. But in the meantime, a lot was happening under the surface—when you couldn't see a thing.

The body grows and changes in spurts. You can see this in children. No one ever sees a child grow. Yet from one year to the next, if the child is measured, there is progress. Your body will grow and change at its own pace. You may see something right away and then nothing for a few weeks or even a month or more. Then suddenly you see progress. Each body is different. The key is not to let your sticking points fool you into thinking nothing is happening. In fact, it is all happening when you see nothing. It's only that it isn't showing up yet. If you stop now, you'll never know what you would have seen. Don't fall into that trap.

Muscle soreness occurs when you have exercised muscles that were previously neglected. It is the result of microscopic tears in the fibers of the ligaments and tendons connecting the muscles, and the slight internal swelling that accompanies these tears. The tears usually occur when you are doing the "elongating" or stretching part of the exercise, when the muscle fibers are lengthening, yet at the same time trying to contract in order to deal with the work being required of them.

These tears are normal and necessary in working out—and the soreness that comes from them is a good sign. The soreness occurs twenty-four to forty-eight hours after the workout. The amount of soreness depends upon how out of shape your muscles are when you start and how hard you work the first time you work out. For example, some women ignore the break-in-gently system, and the day after their workout they can hardly move. But they live to tell about it, and many do not regret it because they feel they needed a rude awakening to realize how out of shape they were.

Never stop working out in the hope that the soreness will go away and never return. Doing this will create an eternal soreness syndrome. You must not skip a workout, but instead, work through the soreness. After about seven minutes of working out, your muscles will feel less stiff, almost as if they've been massaged, due to blood circulation in the muscles.

Muscle injury is quite different from muscle soreness. Injury causes immediate, often sharp, surges of pain. The most common injuries are stretching and tearing ligaments, tears to the fascia (covering of the muscle), and tendinitis (inflammation of a tendon that causes pain). If you follow the exercise instructions and photographs and remember to read the tips, you will have little chance of injury.

If you feel recurring pain and are wondering if it is an injury, play it safe and see your doctor immediately.

Equipment for This Workout

You won't need any! Unless, of course, you choose the option of using weights with your leg routine. You can do this later if you wish, or you can start out with using only one set of weights, say, five-pound dumbbells. You could then switch to the pyramid system—and purchase a set of three-pound weights and a set of eight or ten pounders. But that would be all you would ever need—three sets of dumbbells graduating in weight (I always mean each dumbbell when I refer to pounds of dumbbells). The only time you would need to get more weights would be when your lighter weights become too easy. In this case, for example, you would set aside your three pounders and use fives, eights, and tens. Later you would set aside the fives and use, say, eights, tens, and twelves, and so on, until you reach your maximum. Mine is ten, fifteen, and twenty for thighs.

But again, don't feel obligated to use weights in the beginning. You can do this workout without weights—it's just that you get absolute maximum results with the weights for thighs!

A **dumbbell** is a handheld weight. It is a short metal bar (it can also be made of another material) with raised "ball-type shapes" at either end.

Anatomy of Muscles Used in This Workout

Three muscle groups are exercised in this workout: hips/buttocks, thighs, and abdominals. The following paragraphs will provide a clear description of these muscles so that you can find them on your own body. I want you to place your front- and rear-view photographs next to mine and to label your own body. Then I want you to picture your body evolving into its most perfect form.

The muscles are discussed in the order that they are used in the workout: hips/buttocks, thighs, and abdominals.

HIPS/BUTTOCKS: GLUTEUS MAXIMUS, GLUTEUS MEDIUS, AND GLUTEUS MINIMUS

The gluteus maximus is the largest of the gluteus muscles. It originates from the iliac crest of the thighbone and runs down to the tailbone. It functions to extend and rotate the thigh when significant force is required, such as in stair-climbing. The gluteus medius, located just under the gluteus maximus, functions to raise the leg out to the side and to balance the hips as weight is transferred from one foot to the other. The gluteus minimus originates on the iliac crest of the hipbone and performs the same function as the gluteus maximus.

The above muscles constitute the entire buttocks area, including the side buttocks area, which are the hips and upper outer thigh or "saddlebags." You will notice that certain exercises in this workout specifically zone in on the lower butt, while other focus on the side of the butt (hips or saddlebags), while others cover the entire hips/buttocks area.

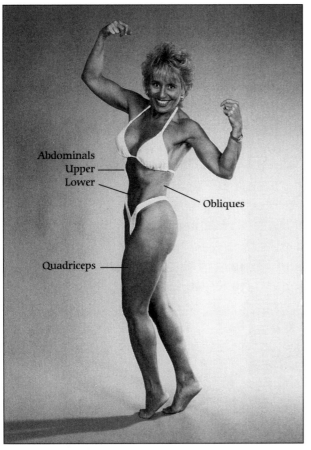

Abdominals
Upper
Lower
Obliques
Quadriceps

Joyce's Front Anatomy

Your Front Anatomy Photo

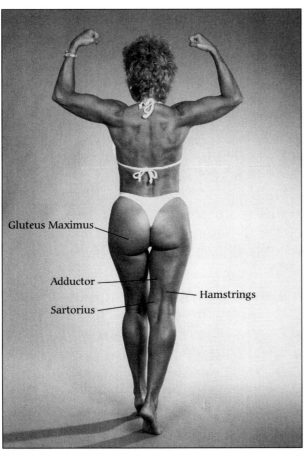

Gluteus Maximus
Adductor
Hamstrings
Sartorius

Joyce's Rear Anatomy
Note: not touched up!

Your Rear Anatomy Photo

FRONT, INNER, AND BACK THIGH: QUADRICEPS, ADDUCTOR, AND
BICEPS FEMORIS OR "HAMSTRINGS"

The front thigh is called the quadriceps muscle. It consists of four muscles, the rectus femoris, and three vasti muscles. These muscles run along the thigh and terminate at the kneecap. These muscles work to extend the leg.

The adductor muscles run along the inner thigh. They originate in the lower pelvic area on the pubic bone and rise to the shaft of the thighbone. This muscle group works in cooperation with other inner thigh muscles to flex, rotate, and pull the legs together from a wide position.

Another inner thigh muscle is the sartorius muscle, the longest muscle in the body. It runs along the inner thigh from the hipbone to the inside of the knee. It functions to rotate the thigh.

The hamstring or biceps femoris muscle group consists of two muscles located on the back thigh. These muscles (the semimembranosus and the semitendinosus) originate in the bony area of the pelvis and terminate at the end of the back of the knee joint. These muscles work to bend the knee.

THE ABDOMINAL MUSCLES: RECTUS ABDOMINAL, EXTERNAL
OBLIQUE, AND INTERNAL OBLIQUE

The rectus abdominus is what we call "the abdominals." But really it is one long, powerful muscle that originates from the fifth through seventh ribs and runs vertically across the abdominal wall. Because this muscle is so long, we often refer to it in sections: Upper abdominals are thought of as being located above the waistline and lower abdominals below the waistline. The abdominal muscles are segmented, so that when developed they can be seen in raised ridgelike form. This development is often referred to as "six-pack" abs.

The abdominal muscles work to pull the upper body toward the lower body. For instance, you use them to sit up from a lying or prone position.

You will notice that certain exercises are specifically designed to challenge the upper abdominals, while other exercises are created to challenge the lower abdominals. However, all abdominal exercises have secondary benefits for the entire abdominal area.

The oblique muscles are located on the side of the body. The external oblique muscles originate at the side of the lower ribs and run diagonally to the rectus abdominus. They are attached to a sheath of fibrous tissue that surrounds the rectus abdominus. These muscles work with other muscles to flex and rotate the torso.

The internal oblique muscles run beneath, and at right angles to, the external oblique muscles. By putting definition in your oblique muscles, you can cause your waist to appear smaller. Once you have lost all excess body fat, the actual size of your waist is determined by the angle of the oblique muscles and cannot be further reduced.

You will notice that certain exercises in this workout are specifically designed to challenge the oblique muscles. As mentioned above, all abdominal exercises have secondary benefits for the entire abdominal area.

Note: Be sure to read each exercise instruction carefully and to be aware of which aspect of the particular muscle is being challenged. Then mentally cooperate by "telling" that aspect of the muscle to do the work and to become tight, toned, developed, and defined.

Workout Plans: Fitting It into Your Real-Life Situation

You have two choices for workout plans: (1) Follow the traditional "split routine" and do this workout every other day, leaving a day of rest between workouts in order to follow the traditional forty-eight-hour recovery principle, or (2) do this workout four to six days a week until you raise your dumbbells for your thigh exercises to fifteen pounds or more, and then go on the split routine. (Note: You can use the split routine using very light weights too!)

You may wonder why I am advising you to ignore the split routine that I have always advocated. First, I must state that only the muscles targeted in this workout can be safely exercised every day. Upper body parts, like the chest, shoulders, biceps, triceps, or back and also the calves, should always be exercised in a split routine. Working them two days in a row could delay your progress and cause muscle atrophy. Why, then, is it okay to break the split routine or forty-eight-hour principle here?

The issue is not the abdominals. You can exercise these muscles two, three, or more days in a row—up to ten days in a row—because the abdominals are not exercised with weights. I never told you this before, but it has always also been okay to exercise the hips/buttocks muscles two or more days in a row because this body part is also not exercised with weights. But it is not absolutely necessary to exercise this area every day. However, if you are in an emergency and want to get into bathing suit shape, you can do it every day.

What about the thigh workout? The thighs are very large muscles and can cope with a daily workout with light weights. If you are using either no weights or very light weights, you can exercise your thighs two or more days in a row. If your goal is to put on significant muscle and if you advance to heavy weights (over fifteen pounds), you must go on the split routine.

One final point: This is a very challenging workout. If you do it every other day, you'll give yourself a day of recuperation in between, not just physically, but also psychologically. If you find yourself feeling burned out by doing it two or more days in a row and begin to dread the workout, immediately switch to the split routine and avoid, at all costs, giving up! Just make sure you do the workout at least three times a week.

WORKOUT PLANS

Plan A. Do the workout every other day.

Plan B. Do the workout four to six days a week.

It's that simple. Instructions on how to incorporate this workout into a total-body workout will be given in Chapter 10.

Get yourself a wall calendar or a daily planner calendar and write your workout days into your appointment schedule. It is, after all, an appointment. An appointment with the most important person in your life: yourself!

When should you work out? You might want to consider doing it first thing in the morning. This way you know for sure it has been done and the day's events will not interfere with your good intentions. Also, working out gives you a boost of energy to start your day. Finally, working out has a great psychological effect. It makes you feel in control. "I did it," you say to yourself. "I have discipline," you think. "I'm a doer," you say. And you forge ahead with a "can do" attitude.

If you can't do your workout in the morning, the next best thing is to find a space at work and do it at lunchtime or on a break. This workout lends itself to a work situation because you don't need any equipment. Lock your office door and do your workout on a towel on the floor. You don't even need a bench.

Your next option is to work out immediately upon returning from work. Do it like a robot; put on your workout clothing and go. It will be over in a matter of minutes.

The most risky time to do your workout is an hour or two after dinner. First, the later you work out, the more chance there is for someone or something to steal your workout time. In addition, for me at least, it's the laziest time of the day. At that time of the evening the last thing in the world I want to do is work out. However, if it were the only available time I had, I would bite the bullet and do it then. No way would I give up working out just because it's inconvenient.

What You Must Forget!

Okay. Now you know what you must remember. It's time to tell what you must forget. Once and for all.

1.   Forget about "devices" or creams that will reshape your thighs, give you a flat "tummy," or melt fat away from your thighs.

Many years ago I bought a device that was supposed to give me thinner thighs. It was an earlier version of one you've seen on TV lately. The instructions said that if I placed the device between my thighs and squeezed, I would get the legs of my dreams. I did exactly as I was told and faithfully worked with the device for the required seven minutes a day. Thirty days later, all I had was a credit card bill; my thighs were as fat, flabby, and shapeless as ever—and every dimple of cellulite was still there.

There are new devices, but the laws of nature have not changed. There are no magical devices that will transform your body. You have to target muscles from a variety of angles with challenging exercises that will eventually reshape, tighten, and define those muscles. No ifs, ands, or buts about it.

The same holds true for thigh fat-remover creams. The creams promise to reduce your thighs by two inches in six weeks. But all they really do is temporarily reduce the size of your thighs by removing excess water weight. The moment you stop applying the cream, your thighs return to their former size. In addition, these creams may well prove dangerous to your health. The skin, as you may already know, is an organ. If you put something on your skin, it is absorbed into your bloodstream.

The bottom line is, creams can't melt fat and make muscle. Only dieting and working out the right way can do that.

2.   Forget about the idea that "after a certain age there's nothing you can do."

I am testimony to the fact that you can reshape your body at any age. I was thirty-eight years old and very fat and out of shape. Look at me now. Thousands of women have sent me their before-and-after photos, showing me that as a result of my workouts they have reshaped their bodies. The vast majority of these women are forty, fifty, sixty, and older. In addition, study after study shows that muscles and bones can be developed at any age—without hours of effort, even at the age of ninety. You can do it at *any* age.

3. Forget about the idea that "it's just genetics. Big hips will always be a nightmare, thunder thighs are in the DNA, and I can't escape my grandmother's potbelly"!

While it is true that your bone structure and tendency toward a certain body shape are built into your DNA, it is *not* true that there's nothing you can do about it. Take what you have and make the best of it. For example, if I did not work on my body, I would have a body exactly like my grandmothers, charming women both, but built like tanks. I decided to chisel my body into its present shape by working out the right way. I would bet my life on it—if my grandmother followed my workout and diet, she would look as good as or better than I do.

4. Forget the lie that cellulite is genetic so there's nothing you can do about it.

As mentioned in Chapter 1, while the tendency toward developing cellulite is genetic, there is indeed something you can do about it. Cellulite is merely bunched-up fat, enlarged fat cells that join together and attach themselves to connecting fibrous tissue just beneath the surface of the skin. This gives the skin an "orange peel" look and feel.

With a low-fat diet and appropriate exercise, in time you can get rid of most, if not all, of your cellulite.

5. Forget the delusion that water pills can help to keep you slim.

Water pills are not the solution to your bloated look and feel. They are simply aids to help when your doctor feels that water retention is causing unnecessary discomfort or hazards to your health. As a general rule, I advise you to stay away from them and to allow your body to level off to a natural amount of water retention. More about this in Chapter 7.

6. Forget the idea that you can't spot-reshape.

True. You can't spot-*reduce* by dieting. After all, you can't tell your body where to lose the fat. But you can spot-change. You can tell your body where to change its shape and feel. You can do it by targeting specific exercises to specific areas on the body.

I've said this before, but I think it bears repeating. Here's how it works: As you hit the muscle from every angle, you gradually chisel the muscle into the desired form. In essence, you completely reshape it, molding it the way a potter works with clay. For example, as you do this workout you will reshape or "spot-change" your hips/buttocks, thighs, and abdominals. This workout will do nothing to reshape your chest, shoulders, biceps, triceps, back, or calves. You would have to do specific exercises for those areas to reshape or spot-change them. So the next time someone says "You can't spot-reduce," tell them you can do more than that. You can completely spot-reshape!

7.   Forget fear of failure.

You've tried so many programs and failed. "Why should I succeed this time?" you ask yourself. I remember a lesson I learned in school. The teacher talked about Thomas Edison, and how many times he failed before he finally came up with a working lightbulb. The teacher constantly reminded us never to give up by asking, "What would have happened if he had given up just one try before he broke through?" So I say to you, this time you will make it. This is a new day—and this is a new workout and you *will* make it this time.

8.   Forget about the tape measure, scale, and fat caliper or other measuring device.

I'm not a bit impressed with measurements, but I am impressed with what I see in living color—in the mirror or in real life. I'll use myself as an example. Plenty of women have smaller dress sizes, weights, and fat percentage measurements than I do—yet they don't look nearly as toned and shapely. Why is this so?

My experience just the other day helps to answer this question. I got into a conversation with a woman in a fitting room of a department store. I noticed that although she was slim, she looked fat. I wondered if she thought she looked good. I asked her if she works out. "No. I just do aerobics," she said, beaming and bragging that she was down to a size 5 dress and weighed only 105 pounds. (She was about five feet two inches.) But the woman had a pouch of fat on her lower stomach and her butt was quite droopy. Her thighs were quite thin but "mushy" looking. I asked her age and she said, "Forty-two, and my body fat is only seventeen percent." "That's great," I said. "Guess how much I weigh?" She guessed 100 pounds. I told her that I weigh 116 and wear a size 3 to 5 dress. She was surprised. "But you must have a very low body fat percentage," she said. "No. I'm about twenty-three percent," I told her. She was astounded. "What's your secret? You look better than I do but your measurements say the opposite." I told her that my secret is my workout. End of story. I couldn't care less what any measuring device says.

9.   Forget about believing that your stretched-out stomach, cellulite-ridden thunder thighs, and wide-load sagging butt are too far gone for remedy. Nothing is impossible with time and effort.

A picture is worth a thousand words. Look at the before-and-after women in Chapter 2. They got great results after working out—for thirty workout hours. You can do it too. Remember, everything comes in time. Next bathing suit season, but for an act of God, you'll still be here. Either you will have more cellulite and look worse than you do now, or you will look better. It all depends upon what you do during that time. So what's it gonna be?

10.   Forget about waiting to lose the weight before you start the workout.

If you wait until you diet down to your weight goal and then start the workout, you will be disgusted with the way your body looks and feels, and you may even be tempted to start eating like a pig again. "I dieted and suffered all this time and this is my reward," you will say. Yes, a flabby, saggy butt, cellulite, loose thighs, and a potbelly. That's what you will have—even at your thinnest—if you don't work out right along with your diet.

Now don't get me wrong. If you do diet first and find yourself a skinny-fat, it is not too late to get the muscle tone to go with your lean body. It is never too late! What I'm saying is that it's quite depressing to see that the diet only reduced your size but did not get you in shape. The answer is clear: The ideal way to go is to do the workout while you are losing the weight! In addition, working out raises your metabolism, so you will actually burn more fat and lose weight faster if you do the workout and develop those muscles (they burn fat twenty-four hours a day, even when you're sleeping).

11.   Forget about shaping your thighs, hips, and butt by stair-stepping.

Stair-stepping machines and step aerobics are good for extra fat burning. In short, they are basically aerobic exercises. To try to use them to sculpt and reshape your hips, butt, and thighs is an exercise in foolishness. It just won't work. These activities do help to strengthen these areas and to build overall endurance, but in order to shape your muscles, you must exercise in a specific manner, in designated "sets" and "repetitions" (and for the thighs, it's a good idea to add weights). In any case, reshaping and defining the body is not a crap shoot where you select an aerobic exercise that seems to target that body part and hope to get lucky. It is a science that has been perfected over the years by champion bodybuilders.

12.   Forget about thinking of working out as a punishment.

All of the research agrees. Exercise is not a punishment. If anything, it is a miracle cure. It strengthens the heart, lowers blood pressure, raises HDL (good cholesterol), lowers blood fats, controls insulin, regulates bowel movements, increases endurance, reduces fatigue, improves muscle tone, and improves your state of mind and even your self-esteem. Finally, it lengthens your life. So if exercise is a punishment, lead me to the jail. I'll glady serve a life sentence!

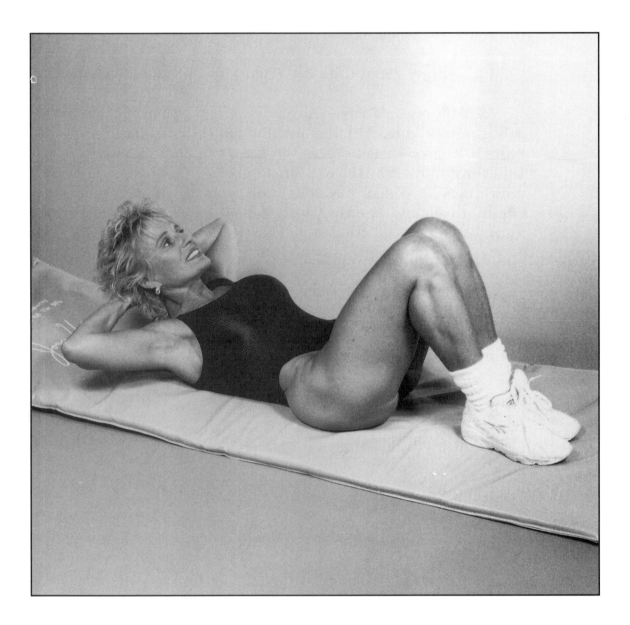

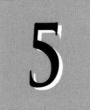

HOW TO DO THE BATHING SUIT WORKOUT

This workout is very simple to learn. In fact, it's the easiest to learn and do of any workout I've invented! You do fifteen repetitions for every single set of every single exercise. You never have to think, "How many reps am I doing now?" In addition, for most exercises, you don't use weights, and for the ones you do, you use only one set of dumbbells (unless you opt to use the pyramid system)—you don't have to worry about switching weights from one set to the next.

In this chapter I'll teach you how to work in tri-sets, the basis for the Bathing Suit Workout. You'll learn the difference between the regular, Iron Woman, Steel Woman, and Titanium Woman workouts. I'll also explain how you can make the workout completely aerobic by eliminating all rests, and how you can make the workout easier and less intense by adding to and/or lengthening the rests.

For those of you who have back or knee problems and/or are extremely overweight and cannot do certain exercises in the workout, I'll tell you how to work out so that you get the full benefit. I'll also discuss how to use the exercise instructions to maximum advantage. Finally, I'll give you a break-in-gently plan, which will take into consideration your present fitness status!

The Regular Bathing Suit Workout

There are seven tri-sets in the regular Bathing Suit Workout. Each tri-set consists of one exercise each for hips/buttocks, thighs, and abdominals. They are:

HIPS/BUTTOCKS	THIGHS	ABDOMINALS
1. Saddlebag stripper crunch	Lying inner thigh lift	Knee-raised oblique
2. Lower butt curl	Leg curl	Bent-knee sewn lift
3. Lower butt crunch	Chair position firmer	Knee-raised crunch
4. Lower butt side kick	Straddle squat	Side oblique crunch
5. Floor feather kick-up	Front squat	Ceiling sewn lift
6. Lying butt lift	Lunge	Toe-reach crunch
7. One-leg prone butt lift	Regular squat	Ceiling oblique reach

How to Do the Bathing Suit Workout: Working in Tri-Sets

A tri-set is a combination of three compatible exercises that is done without taking a rest. Only after one set of exercise has been performed for each of those three body parts can a fifteen-second rest be taken.

REPETITIONS AND SETS

You will do fifteen repetitions for each set of every single exercise in this workout. It's that simple. But there's a catch, albeit an easy one. Instead of working in normal sets where you rest after each set, you will work in triple sets or tri-sets, where you do a set for three different exercises before you take a rest.

WEIGHTS

You have the option of using a set of five-pound dumbbells for thigh exercises only. You will be reminded of this in the exercise instructions. In time, as the five-pound dumbbells become too easy, raise your weights to eight or ten pounds. When those weights get too easy, go to twelve or fifteen pounds—even twenty! If you choose to do so, you could "pyramid" your thighs, using the modified pyramid system described on pp. 32–33. In this case you will need three sets of dumbbells: threes, fives, and tens. You may also use an optional three- or five-pound dumbbell for any appropriate abdominal exercise.

STRETCHING

If you wish, do one to three relaxed repetitions of each exercise in the entire workout before you start or do your favorite set of stretches.

HOW DO THE TRI-SETS WORK?

Let's take a look at exactly how it works by looking at the first tri-set of the workout.

HIPS/BUTTOCKS	THIGHS	ABDOMINALS
1. Saddlebag stripper	Lying inner thigh lift	Knee-raised oblique crunch

Here's how you proceed:

You do one set of fifteen repetitions of the first hips/buttocks exercise, the saddlebag stripper. Without resting, you do one set of fifteen repetitions of the first thigh exercise, the lying inner thigh lift. Again, without resting, you do one set of fifteen repetitions the first abdominal exercise, the knee-raised oblique crunch.

Whew. Now you take a fifteen-second rest.

Back to work. You repeat exactly what you just did one more time.

Now you can take another hard-earned fifteen-second rest. Now move to the third and final set. You repeat exactly what you did your third and final time.

Now you take a fifteen-second rest, and move to your second tri-set.

HIPS/BUTTOCKS	THIGHS	ABDOMINALS
2. Lower butt curl	Leg curl	Bent-knee sewn lift

You do one set of fifteen repetitions of the second hips/buttocks exercise, the lower butt curl. Without resting, you do one set of fifteen repetitions of the second thigh exercise, the leg curl. Again, without resting, you do one set of fifteen repetitions of the second abdominal exercise, the bent-knee sewn lift.

Now you can take a fifteen-second rest.

Back to work. You repeat exactly what you just did one more time.

Take another fifteen-second rest. Then move to the final set and repeat exactly what you did before for the last time.

Take a fifteen-second rest and move to your third group of exercises.

HIPS/BUTTOCKS	THIGHS	ABDOMINALS
3. Lower butt crunch	Chair position firmer	Knee-raised crunch

You do one set of fifteen repetitions of the third hips/buttocks exercise, the lower butt crunch. Without resting, you do one set of fifteen repetitions of the third thigh exercise, chair position firmer. Again, without resting, you do one set of fifteen repetitions the third abdominal exercise, the knee-raised crunch.

Now you can take a fifteen-second rest.

Back to work. You repeat exactly what you just did one more time.

Take another fifteen-second rest. Then move to the third and final tri-set and repeat exactly what you did before for the last time.

Take a fifteen-second rest and move to your fourth group of exercises. Continue to work as above until you have completed all seven tri-sets.

SETS, REPETITIONS, AND RESTS IN ABBREVIATED FORM

Now let's take a look at the sets, repetitions, and rests as they will apply to all tri-sets in this workout.

> Tri-Set 1: Fifteen repetitions each without resting: hips/buttocks exercise, thigh exercise, abdominal exercise. Rest fifteen seconds.
>
> Tri-Set 2: Fifteen repetitions each without resting: hips/buttocks exercise, thigh exercise, abdominal exercise. Rest fifteen seconds.
>
> Tri-Set 3: Fifteen repetitions each without resting: hips/buttocks exercise, thigh exercise, abdominal exercise. Rest fifteen seconds.

Move to the next tri-set. Repeat as above until all seven tri-sets are completed.

The Iron Woman Workout

You work exactly as above. The only difference is that instead of stopping after you've done your seven tri-sets, you do an eighth tri-set. Your workout will look like this.

HIPS/BUTTOCKS	THIGHS	ABDOMINALS
1. Saddlebag stripper	Lying inner thigh lift	Knee-raised oblique crunch
2. Lower butt curl	Leg curl	Bent-knee sewn lift
3. Lower butt crunch	Chair position firmer	Knee-raised crunch
4. Lower butt side kick	Straddle squat	Side oblique crunch
5. Floor feather kick-up	Front squat	Ceiling sewn lift
6. Lying butt lift	Lunge	Toe-reach crunch
7. One-leg prone butt lift	Regular squat	Ceiling oblique reach
8. Standing butt squeeze	Hack squat	Knee-in

The Steel Woman Workout

You work exactly as above. The only difference is that, instead of stopping after you've done eight tri-sets, you do a ninth tri-set. Your workout will look like this:

HIPS/BUTTOCKS	THIGHS	ABDOMINALS
1. Saddlebag stripper	Lying inner thigh lift	Knee-raised oblique crunch
2. Lower butt curl	Leg curl	Bent-knee sewn lift
3. Lower butt crunch	Chair position firmer	Knee-raised crunch
4. Lower butt side kick	Straddle squat	Side oblique crunch
5. Floor feather kick-up	Front squat	Ceiling sewn lift
6. Lying butt lift	Lunge	Toe-reach crunch
7. One-leg prone butt lift	Regular squat	Ceiling oblique reach
8. Standing butt squeeze	Hack squat	Knee-in
9. Reverse-lunge lift	Bent-knee deadlift	Sit-up

The Titanium Woman Workout

You work exactly as above. The only difference is that, instead of stopping after you've done nine tri-sets, you do a tenth tri-set. Your workout will look like this:

HIPS/BUTTOCKS	THIGHS	ABDOMINALS
1. Saddlebag stripper	Lying inner thigh lift	Knee-raised oblique crunch
2. Lower butt curl	Leg curl	Bent-knee sewn lift
3. Lower butt crunch	Chair position firmer	Knee-raised crunch
4. Lower butt side kick	Straddle squat	Side oblique crunch
5. Floor feather kick-up	Front squat	Ceiling sewn lift
6. Lying butt lift	Lunge	Toe-reach crunch
7. One-leg prone butt lift	Regular squat	Ceiling oblique reach
8. Standing butt squeeze	Hack squat	Knee-in
9. Reverse-lunge lift	Bent-knee deadlift	Sit-up
10. Straight leg kick-up	Sissy squat	Leg raise

Review

Whether you are doing the regular, Iron Woman, Steel Woman, or Titanium Woman workout, you work in the same manner. You do one set of three different exercises for three different body parts before you take a rest: hips/buttocks, thighs, and abdominals. You can get an overview of your particular workout by looking at the above lists. If you look across the numbers horizontally, you will clearly see your tri-sets.

Don't worry. You don't have to remember anything. I lead you along in the exercise section. Each exercise is placed after the other, in the order that they are done. And so you won't have to keep turning pages, you can use the handy tear-out wall chart on pp. 209–230. This chart shows you a mini-overview of all of your exercises in reduced photographs.

Make the Workout Completely Aerobic by Eliminating All the Rests

After you've been doing the workout for a while, you may find that you can skip most or all of the rests. If you do that, you will have a completely aerobic workout. In addition, you will save time.

Make the Workout Easier and Less Intense by Adding and/or Lengthening Rests

This is a very demanding workout. Even after breaking in gently, you may feel that the workout is too much for you and may be tempted to quit. Don't do it! Instead, add one or more of the following techniques.

1. Take a fifteen-second rest after *each* set. This means that, instead of doing strict tri-sets where you don't rest until you've completed one set for each of three exercises, you would do gentle tri-sets where you rest fifteen seconds after each set. This would triple your rest periods. The workout would take longer, but it may enable you to go on, whereas before you might have given up in discouragement. If you work this way, you will still get the full body-sculpting, muscle-defining benefit. All you will lose will be some of the aerobic effect.

If that's not enough you can add in #2.

2. Do as above, only double the rest time. Take thirty-second rests between each set. If that's not enough you can add in #3.

3. Do as described in 1 and 2, only reduce the number of tri-sets. Pick out the four tri-sets that are easiest for you to do, and do only those tri-sets.

If you choose one of the above plans, in time you may or may not decide to shorten your rests and eliminate some of them, and add exercises, so that you will eventually be doing the full-force workout. If not, you will still derive a great deal of benefit from the workout.

If You Are Extremely Overweight, Out of Shape, or Cannot Do Certain, Even Many, Exercises

Some of you may open the book with all good intentions, but after trying a certain exercise say to yourselves, "Forget it. I'll never be able to do this." Instead of quitting outright, go through the workout and see which exercises you *can* do. Do only those exercises by substituting them for exercises you can't do. All you have to do is remember to pick an exercise from the same body part and double up. Let me explain.

Suppose you have zipped through your first three groups of exercises. You've done the saddlebag stripper, the lying inner thigh lift, and the knee-raised oblique crunch; the lower butt curl, the leg curl, and the bent-knee sewn lift; and the lower butt crunch, the chair position firmer, and the knee-raised crunch. You are up to your fourth group of exercises. You do the first exercise in that tri-set, the lower butt side kick. But when you come to your second exercise, the straddle squat, you can't do it because you have bad knees. You can't squat at all. Simple. Look back at all the exercises for that body part, in this case the thighs, and pick an exercise from that body part that you can do and do it in place of the difficult exercise. For example, you may have found the lying inner thigh lift that you did in tri-set number one manageable. So do it again, in place of the straddle squat.

Let's continue the example. Now you're going along in your workout, but soon you get to the lunge. You can't do that. Okay. Pick another thigh exercise that you could do. Maybe the leg curl. You continue on, and sure enough, there's another exercise you can't do. The front frog squat. So you double up on the chair position firmer. And so on.

This will hold true with any exercise. If you can't do it, the rule of thumb is to pick one from the same body part and double up on it. You have ten exercises to choose from.

If your knees or back are really bad, you may find yourself tripling up on some exercises. There may be only four that you can cope with. Fine. You'll still get the major benefit of the workout. You just won't be hitting the muscle from as many angles, that's all.

How to Take Full Advantage of the Exercise Instructions

The first thing you'll see in the exercise instructions is the number of the tri-set and the names of the three exercises in that tri-set. Next you'll see the name of the particular exercise that you will do, and a description of the muscles that will be shaped and defined by that exercise.

Next you'll see the word "Position." Here you'll get a detailed description of how to place yourself in order to start the workout. However, a picture is worth a thousand words, so look at the "Start" photograph first and then as you study the photograph, read the "Position" instructions to be sure that you don't miss anything. For example, you may note that I tell you to press your back into the mat, or to raise your head slightly off the floor, and so on. This may not be obviously visible in the photographs until it is pointed out.

Next you'll see the heading "Movement." The finish photograph depicts where you will have "moved to." Look at that first and then read the "Movement" instructions. They tell you exactly how to execute the exercise. You'll want to look at both the start and finish photographs as you read this section and imagine yourself doing the exercise. Go through it in your mind exactly as if you are doing it.

Next comes "Tips." This is very important section. I know the tendencies of beginning exercisers to make certain mistakes, and I've made a special effort to head you off before you fall into the common traps. For example, I remind you not to pull on your neck when doing a crunch, or to stretch gently into a side oblique crunch rather than force it, or to keep your mind riveted on a working muscle, or not to hold your breath, and so on.

Finally, there is the "Machines, etc." section. Here you will be given alternatives. Sometimes I'll suggest a barbell, other times a machine, and other times an alternative exercise. You could completely ignore this section if you want to, or you can use it for variety.

Before you actually start your workout, it's a good idea to read through the exercise instructions, looking at the photographs and trying to do one repetition of each exercise. Do this just to feel it out in your mind, on a day when you are going through the book in a relaxed mood. This is also a great way to precondition yourself for the actual workout. Then set a date to start the break-in-gently system.

Breaking In Gently if You Are in Aerobic Shape and Have Been Doing One of My Other Workouts

Good news. You can do the full regular workout if you can cope with it. If not, switch to one of the other break-in-gently plans.

Week 1. Full Regular Workout.

If you are planning to do the Iron Woman, Steel Woman, or Titanium Woman workouts, add them in one week at a time!

Breaking In Gently if You Are in Aerobic Shape but Have Never Done One of My Workouts

Week 1. One tri-set of the first seven exercises (the regular workout). Do only as many of the fifteen repetitions for each set as you can do.

Week 2. Two tri-sets of the first seven exercises (the regular workout). Do only as many of the fifteen repetitions for each set as you can do.

Week 3. Three tri-sets of the first seven exercises (the regular workout). Do only as many of the fifteen repetitions for each set as you can do.

Weeks 4–6 or more. Now you are on the full program. Keep working until you can do three sets of fifteen repetitions for all three exercises of all seven tri-sets. Then, if you wish, you can add the Iron, Steel, and/or Titanium Woman workouts to your schedule, one week at a time.

Breaking In Gently if You Have Done One of My Workouts Before but You Are Not in Aerobic Shape

Week 1. Do one tri-set of each of the first seven exercises, only "cheat" by taking a fifteen-second rest after each set.

Week 2. Do one tri-set of the first seven exercises without cheating.

Week 3. Try to do two tri-sets of the first seven exercises without cheating, but take an extra rest when you must.

Week 4. Do two tri-sets of the first seven exercises without cheating.

Week 5. Try to do all three sets of the first seven exercises without cheating, but take an extra rest when you must.

Weeks 6–8 or more. Do all three tri-sets of the first seven exercises without cheating. Wait until you are doing full fifteen-repetition tri-sets and then, if you wish, one week at a time, add on exercises until you are doing the Titanium Woman workout.

Note: Don't hold yourself back. Advance more quickly if you can. This is just a guideline.

Breaking In Gently if You Are Extremely Overweight and/or Out of Shape Period

You're in bad shape. You're very out of shape and/or very fat, very weak, and extremely out of breath when you try to do the workout.

You think, "Forget it. I'll never be able to do this." Think again. Here's the way to go.

Look at the exercise photographs and pick out any tri-set that you can do. Then pick another and another, until you have made up four tri-sets. If you can't do it that way, re-create the tri-sets by picking out all the hips/buttocks exercises you can do, all the thigh exercises you can do, and all the abdominal exercises you can do. Then arrange those exercises into new tri-sets that suit you. If you are short on one exercise for a tri-set, double up as described above. Once you have your four tri-sets, you may want to photocopy the photographs and arrange them in the order that you will be doing them.

Now here's how to proceed:

Week 1. Sets one to three of one tri-set, three repetitions each. Cheat and rest between each tri-set.

Week 2. Sets one to three of one tri-set, six repetitions each. Cheat and rest between each tri-set.

Week 3. Sets one to three of one tri-set, nine repetitions each. Cheat and rest between each tri-set.

Week 4. Sets one to three of one tri-set, twelve repetitions each. Cheat and rest between each tri-set.

Week 5. Sets one to three of one tri-set, fifteen repetitions each. Cheat and rest between each tri-set.

Week 6. Sets one to three of one tri-set, fifteen repetitions each. No cheating.

Week 7–on. You will add your second tri-set slowly, exactly as above. In six more weeks you will be doing two full tri-sets. You will now have been working out for twelve weeks. Then you will add in your third tri-set, exactly as above. In eighteen weeks you will be doing three full tri-sets. Again, you will add in your fourth tri-set exactly as above. In twenty-four weeks you will be doing four full tri-sets. Just keep going in the same manner as above until you are on the full program and I suspect you will!

You may find that you can advance more quickly than the above schedule. If so, fine. Go at your own pace. In addition, you may find that indeed you can now do some of the exercises that previously seemed impossible. Great. Add them in. If you persist, in time you will be able to do seven full tri-sets.

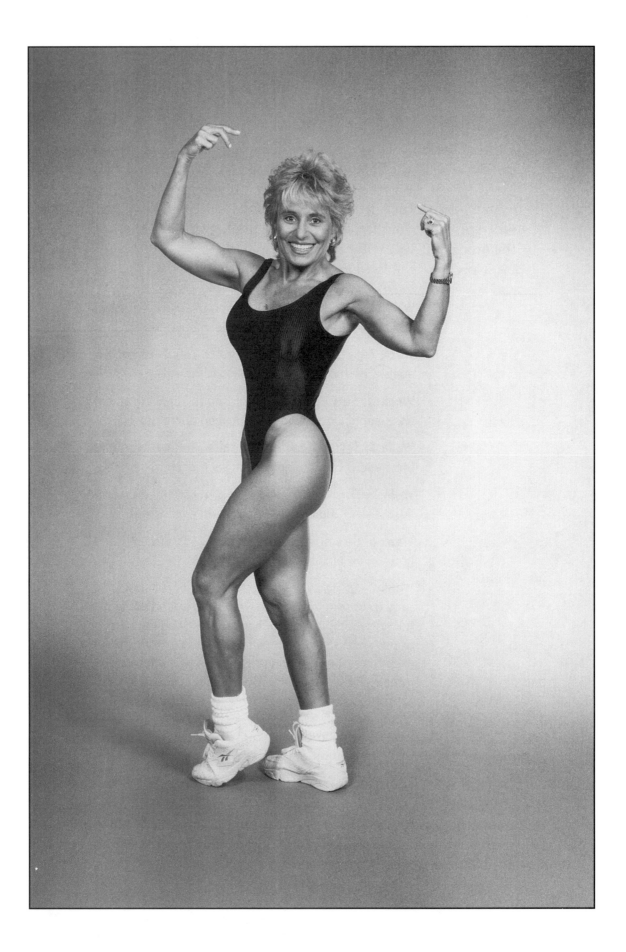

6

THE BATHING SUIT WORKOUT

Now you are ready to do the workout. Remember, you do fifteen repetitions for each set of each exercise. The only exercises that will allow optional weights are most of the thigh exercises, in which case you will use five-pound dumbbells (or less or more weight, depending upon how strong you are and if you decide to pyramid), and one hips/buttocks exercise. All other exercises are done without weights.

You will be exercising in tri-sets, busting the bulge that circles your middle and transforming it into a triangle of tight, toned muscle. You will always start with hips/buttocks, then move to thighs, and end with abdominals. Then you'll take an optional fifteen-second rest and move to the next tri-set.

If you are doing the regular workout, you'll do the first seven tri-sets. If you're performing the Iron Woman workout, you'll work through the first eight tri-sets. If you're conquering the Steel Woman workout, you'll continue through the first nine cycles. If you are challenging yourself with the ultimate conquest, the Titanium Woman workout, you'll complete all ten tri-sets.

If you want to do all ten cycles but find that some of the exercises are too difficult, as mentioned before, choose any exercise from the same body part that you *can* do, and simply substitute that exercise for the one you can't do.

This is not a game. It's not for people who want to make themselves think they have worked out but in reality have done little more than move around a bit. It's a surefire system to get rid of the fat and produce definition and muscle. It *is* work, but you can't put a price on the permanent prize you will get for your effort!

1

SADDLEBAG STRIPPER, LYING INNER THIGH LIFT, AND KNEE-RAISED OBLIQUE CRUNCH

HIPS/BUTTOCKS: SADDLEBAG STRIPPER SLIMS AND TONES THE "SADDLEBAG" HIP AREA.

POSITION   Lie on the floor on your side supporting yourself with your elbow, your hand behind your head. Cross your other arm in front of you and place the palm of that hand on the floor, in front of your chest, as a brace. Bend your lower (nonworking) leg. One side of your body will be completely aligned on the floor.

MOVEMENT   With your hips aligned and keeping your working knee facing front, flexing your working hip/buttock area as you go, raise your upper leg as high as possible. Return to the start position and repeat the movement until you have finished your set. Perform the set for the other side of your body. Without resting, move to the next exercise in this tri-set, the lying inner thigh lift.

TIPS   Keep your hips aligned as you work. Don't let your body tilt over to the back or the front. Your hips should be "stacked," one lying on the top of the other. Don't hold or think about your breath. Breathe naturally.

MACHINES, ETC. You may substitute this exercise for any hip abductor machine at twenty pounds.

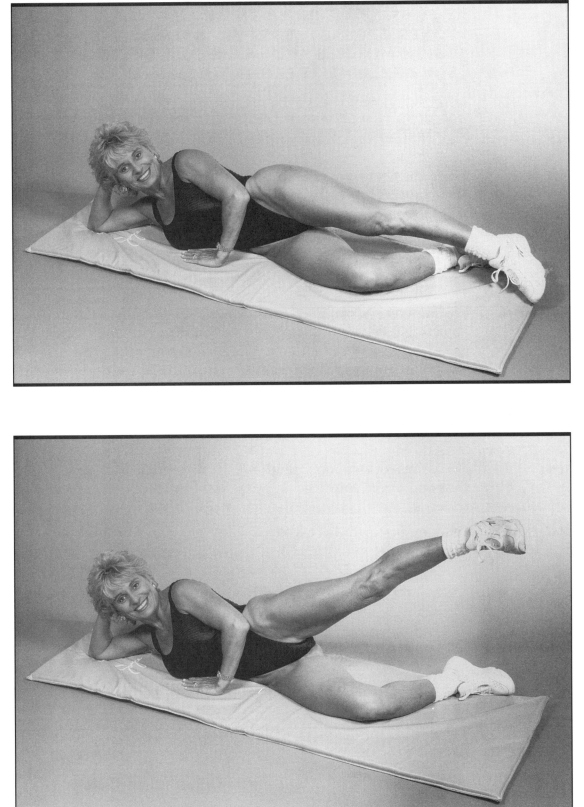

THIGHS: LYING INNER THIGH LIFT TIGHTENS, TONES, STRENGTHENS, AND DEFINES THE INNER THIGH MUSCLES AND HELPS TO TIGHTEN AND TONE THE ENTIRE FRONT THIGH MUSCLE.

NOTE: THIS EXERCISE HAS BEEN CALLED "SIDE LEG LIFT" IN OTHER WORKOUTS. I HAVE CHANGED THE NAME TO MAKE IT MORE DESCRIPTIVE OF THE ACTUAL EXERCISE.

POSITION   Lie on the floor on your side, supporting yourself with your elbow. Bend your upper (nonworking) leg at the knee and place the sole of that foot on the ground. One side of your body should be completely aligned on the floor. Extend your lower (working) leg and place a dumbbell in the middle of your thigh area. Hold it there with your free hand as you work.

MOVEMENT   Keeping your working leg extended and holding the weight on your thigh, flex your inner thigh as you lift your entire leg off the ground until you cannot go any higher. Keeping the pressure on your working inner thigh muscle, return to the start position, and repeat the movement until you have completed your set. Repeat the set for the other side of your body. Without resting, move to the final exercise in this tri-set, the knee-raised oblique crunch.

TIPS   Flex your working inner thigh muscle as hard as possible as you raise and lower your leg.

MACHINES, ETC.   You may perform this exercise on any hip adductor machine at twenty pounds.

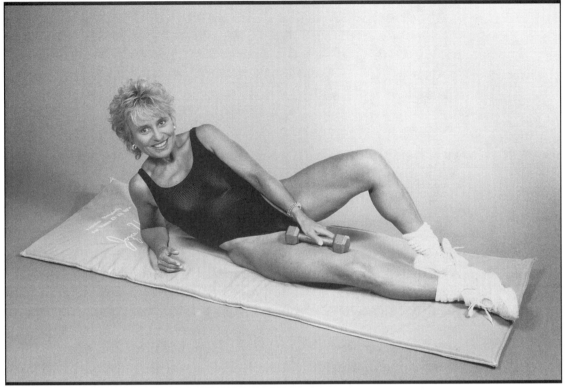

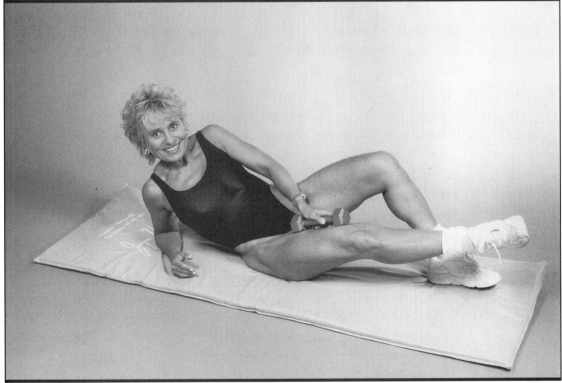

THE BATHING SUIT WORKOUT | **67**

ABDOMINALS: KNEE-RAISED OBLIQUE CRUNCH STRENGTHENS, TIGHTENS, TONES, AND DEFINES THE OBLIQUE AND UPPER ABDOMINAL MUSCLES, AND HELPS TO TIGHTEN THE LOWER ABDOMINAL AREA.

POSITION   Lie flat on the floor with your knees raised and your legs crossed at the ankles. Place your hands behind your head.

MOVEMENT   Leading with your chin, raise your left shoulder off the floor while at the same time bringing your right elbow to your right inner knee, all the time flexing your abdominal muscles. In full control, return to the start position and repeat the movement for the other side of your body. Continue this alternating twisting-crunch movement until you have completed your set. Rest an optional fifteen seconds and do another tri-set of this combination. Again, take an optional fifteen-second rest and perform the third and final tri-set of this combination. Rest an optional fifteen seconds more and proceed to the first exercise of the next tri-set, the lower butt curl.

TIPS   Don't jerk your body as you try to get your elbow to reach the opposite inner-knee area. Feel the flex in your oblique muscles as you go into the oblique crunch position, and enjoy the stretch on the back-to-start position.

MACHINES, ETC.   You may perform this exercise on any rotary torso machine.

Now that you can do all three exercises, let's get down to business.

WHAT TO DO: Set 1: Fifteen repetitions each: saddlebag stripper, lying inner thigh
TRI-SETS,   lift, knee-raised oblique crunch. Optional fifteen-second rest.
REPETITIONS,   Set 2: Fifteen repetitions each: saddlebag stripper, lying inner thigh
WEIGHTS   lift, knee-raised oblique crunch. Optional fifteen-second rest.
Set 3: Fifteen repetitions each: saddlebag stripper, lying inner thigh lift, knee-raised oblique crunch. Optional fifteen-second rest.

NOTE: You can use five-pound dumbbells for lying inner thigh lift, or you can pyramid. No weights used for other exercises. If you choose to use the modified pyramid system for thigh work, see pp. 32–33 for a review.

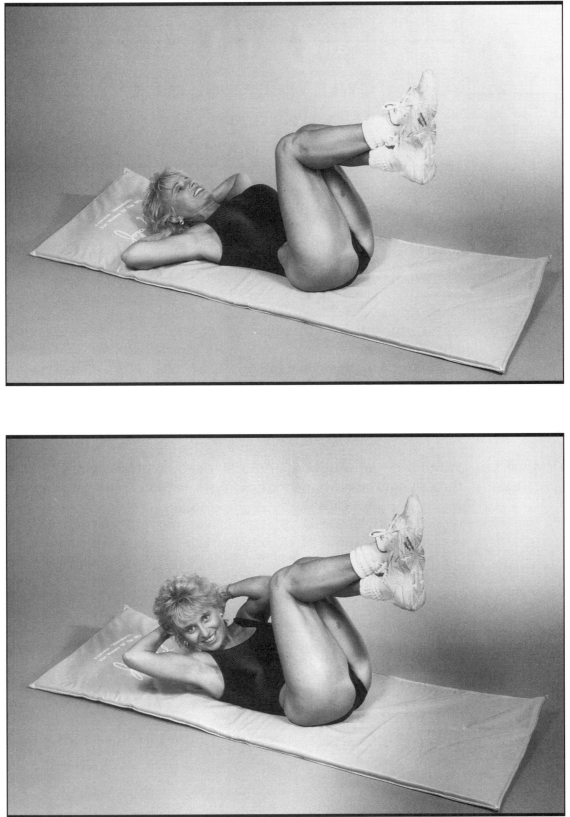

THE BATHING SUIT WORKOUT | **69**

2

LOWER BUTT CURL, LEG CURL, AND BENT-KNEE SEWN LIFT

HIPS/BUTTOCKS: LOWER BUTT CURL TIGHTENS, TONES, LIFTS, AND SHAPES THE LOWER BUTT AREA AND HELPS TO REDUCE SADDLEBAGS.

POSITION   Lie on your side with your lower leg bent back and your upper leg extended in line with your body. Your hips should be "stacked," in line with each other. Lean on your lower elbow for support and place that hand behind your head. Cross your upper arm in front of your chest and place the palm of that hand on the floor for support.

MOVEMENT   Without tilting your body (your hips should remain aligned throughout the movement), bending at the knee, curl your upper leg toward your chest as far as you can go. Feel the stretch in your working buttock muscle. Flex your working buttock muscle as you go, and in full control. Return to start. Repeat the movement until you have completed your set. Repeat the set for the other side of your body. Without resting, move to the next exercise in this tri-set, the leg curl.

TIPS   Don't merely go through the motions, sloppily curling your leg in half-hearted movements. Instead, focus on your working buttock muscle and flex as hard as possible on the return movement. Don't hold your breath. Breathe naturally.

MACHINES, ETC. You may perform this exercise on any butt-curl machine. Set the weight at twenty pounds.

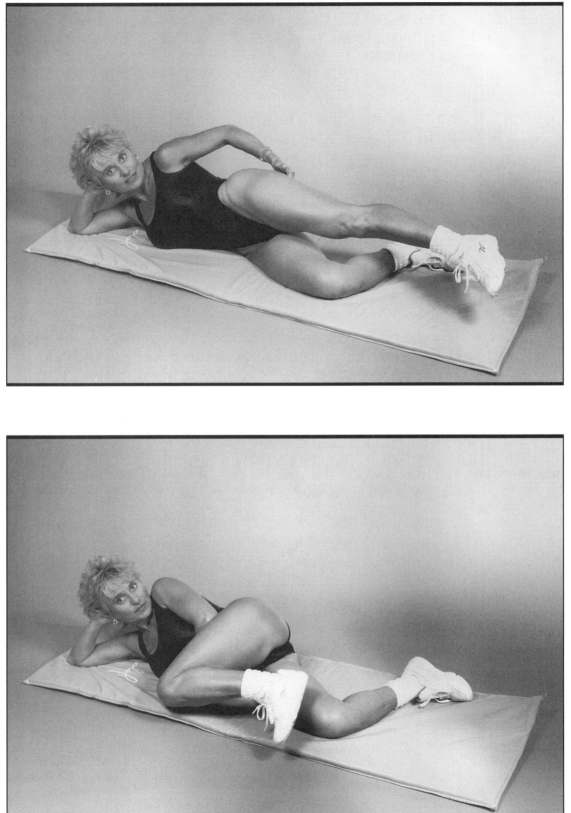

THIGHS: LEG CURL TIGHTENS, TONES, SHAPES, AND DEFINES THE BACK THIGH MUSCLES (HAMSTRINGS).

POSITION   With a dumbbell placed between your feet, lie in a prone position on the floor or on a flat exercise bench. Extend your legs straight out behind you and lean on your elbows for support.

MOVEMENT   Bending at the knees and flexing your back thigh muscles as you go, raise your legs until they are perpendicular to the floor. Keeping the pressure on your back thigh muscles as hard as possible, return to the start position and repeat the movement until you have completed your set. Without resting, proceed to the final exercise in this tri-set, the bent-knee sewn lift.

TIPS   If you squeeze your ankles together, you will better be able to keep the pressure on your back thigh muscles. Don't do this exercise without sneakers, and especially not barefoot. You'll hurt your feet—and if you are using a dumbbell, it may slip! Don't swing the dumbbell up and down. Maintain control throughout the movement.

MACHINES, ETC. You may perform this exercise on any leg-curl machine. Set the weight at twenty pounds.

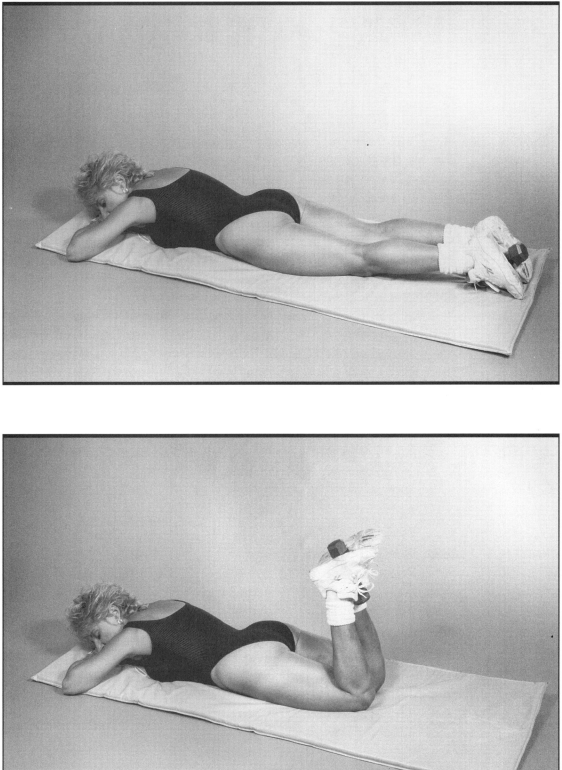

THE BATHING SUIT WORKOUT | **73**

ABDOMINALS: BENT-KNEE SEWN LIFT
TIGHTENS, TONES, STRENGTHENS, AND DEFINES
THE ENTIRE LOWER ABDOMINAL AREA AND HELPS
TO STRENGTHEN THE LOWER BACK.

POSITION

Lie on the floor and place your hands behind your head. Raise your legs off the floor, bending at the knee and crossing your feet at the ankles. Push your back into the floor so that there is no "curve" or space in your back.

MOVEMENT

Making believe that your belly button is sewn to the ground, lift your buttocks off the floor about two to three inches, while at the same time flexing your lower abdominal muscles as hard as possible. (Remember, you couldn't go much higher even if you tried. Your belly button is sewn to the ground.) Repeat this movement until you have completed your set. Rest an optional fifteen seconds and do another tri-set of this combination. Again, take an optional fifteen-second rest and perform the third and final tri-set of this combination. Rest an optional fifteen seconds more and proceed to the first exercise of the next tri-set, the lower butt crunch.

MACHINES, ETC.

You may substitute this exercise for the standard knee-in as demonstrated in my book *Bottoms Up!*

WHAT TO DO:
TRI-SETS,
REPETITIONS,
WEIGHTS

Set 1: Fifteen repetitions each: lower butt curl, leg curl, bent-knee sewn lift. Optional fifteen-second rest.

Set 2: Fifteen repetitions each: lower butt curl, leg curl, bent-knee sewn lift. Optional fifteen-second rest.

Set 3: Fifteen repetitions each: lower butt curl, leg curl, bent-knee sewn lift. Optional fifteen-second rest.

NOTE:

Use five-pound dumbbells for leg curl (optional). No weights required for other exercises. If you choose to use the modified pyramid system for your thighs, see p. 33 for review.

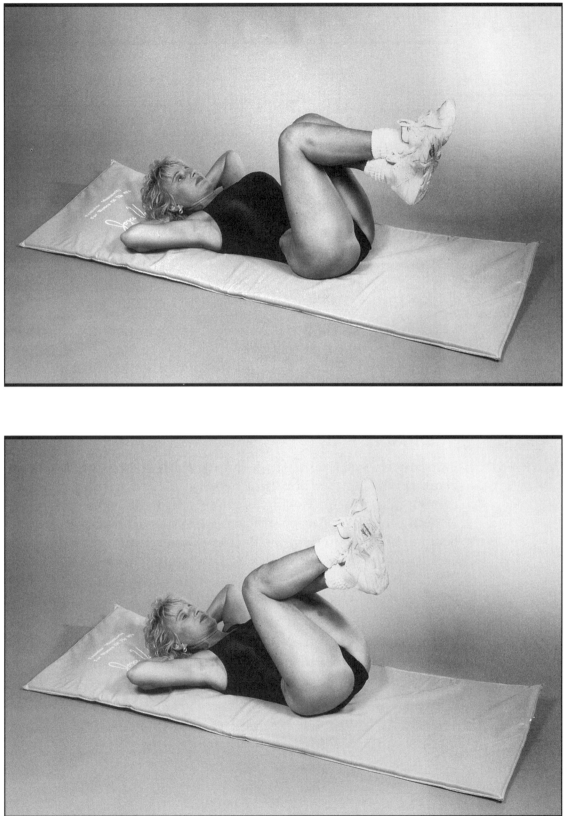

3

LOWER BUTT CRUNCH, CHAIR POSITION FIRMER, AND KNEE-RAISED CRUNCH

HIPS/BUTTOCKS: LOWER BUTT CRUNCH LIFTS, TIGHTENS, TONES, AND SHAPES THE LOWER BUTT AREA.

POSITION   With your hands clasped behind your head, lie flat on your back. Raise your legs so that they are vertical to the floor and flex your feet toward your body. Lift your head and shoulders slightly off the floor (as if you are doing a crunch). Keeping one leg straight, bend the knee of the other leg until the heel of the foot of your bent leg touches your ankle, or at least the ankle area.

MOVEMENT   Flexing your working buttock muscle as you go, straighten your bent leg while at the same time bending the other leg in a stair-climbing movement. Flexing as you go, straighten the newly bent leg and bend the other leg. Continue this alternate straightening-bending motion, all the time flexing your working buttock muscles as hard as possible, until you have completed a set for each side of your body. Without resting, move to the next exercise in this tri-set, the chair position firmer.

TIPS   Keep your back flat on the floor throughout the movement. Give your working buttock an extra-hard flex at the point where you unbend your leg.

MACHINES, ETC. You may substitute this exercise for a butt curl machine.

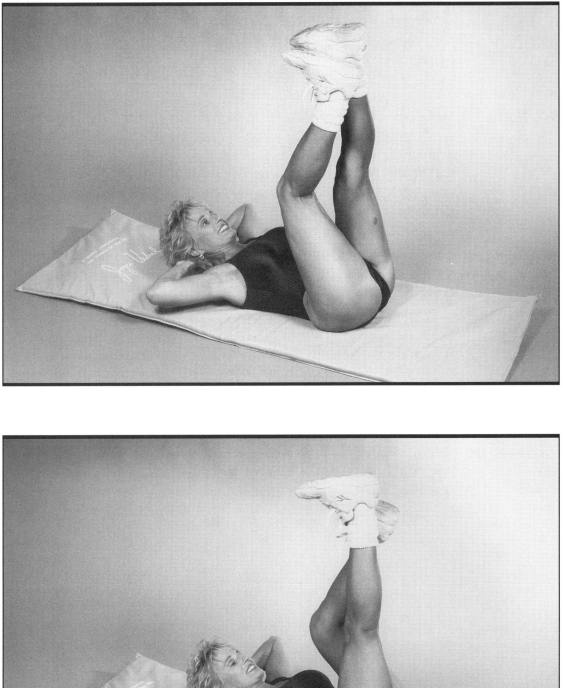

THIGHS: CHAIR POSITION FIRMER TIGHTENS, TONES, AND STRENGTHENS THE FRONT THIGHS AND HIPS.

POSITION Make believe you are sitting in a chair that is placed against a wall—only do it without a chair! (See photo.) Your back will be flat against the wall, your legs will form a right angle, and your feet will be flat on the floor. Place the optional dumbbells on each knee and gently hold them. If you are not using weights, place your hands on your knees.

MOVEMENT Good news. Do nothing. Count for fifteen seconds and, without resting, move to the final exercise in this tri-set, the knee-raised crunch.

TIPS Don't fall into the trap of holding your breath. Breathe naturally. For additional benefit, flex your front thighs as hard as possible for the full fifteen seconds. Also, if you wish, later you can raise the amount of time to as long as a full minute! This is completely optional.

MACHINES, ETC. You may substitute this exercise for an exercise done on any hips/buttocks machine. Choose a comfortable starting weight. Machines vary, so you'll have to experiment.

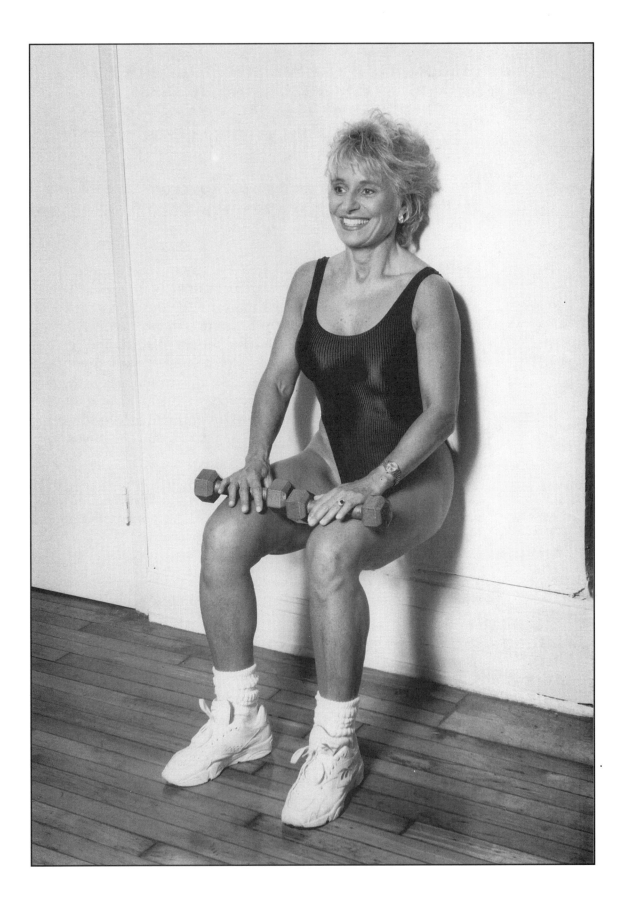

ABDOMINALS: KNEE-RAISED CRUNCH DEVELOPS, SHAPES, STRENGTHENS, AND DEFINES THE ENTIRE UPPER ABDOMINAL AREA AND HELPS TO STRENGTHEN THE LOWER ABDOMINAL AREA.

POSITION

Lie flat on your back on the floor, pull your knees up until your legs form an **L**, and cross your feet at the ankles. Place your hands behind your head.

MOVEMENT

Flexing your entire abdominal area as you go, raise your shoulders off the floor in a curling movement until your shoulders are completely off the floor, all the time keeping your knees raised so that your legs are still in an approximate **L** shape. Keeping the pressure on your abdominal muscles, return to start, and repeat the movement until you have completed your set. Rest an optional fifteen seconds and do another tri-set of this combination. Again, take an optional fifteen-second rest and perform the third and final tri-set of this combination. Rest an optional fifteen seconds and proceed to the first exercise of the next tri-set, the lower butt side kick.

TIPS

Don't allow yourself to use your hands behind your head to pull yourself up. You'll hurt your neck. Instead, let your upper abdominals do the work.

MACHINES, ETC.

You may substitute this exercise with any crunch machine, or with the standard sit-up as demonstrated in my book *Gut Busters*.

WHAT TO DO: TRI-SETS, REPETITIONS, WEIGHTS

Set 1: Fifteen repetitions each: lower butt crunch, chair position firmer, knee-raised crunch. Optional fifteen-second rest.
Set 2: Fifteen repetitions each: lower butt crunch, chair position firmer, knee-raised crunch. Optional fifteen-second rest.
Set 3: Fifteen repetitions each: lower butt crunch, chair position firmer, knee-raised crunch. Optional fifteen-second rest.

NOTE:

You may place an optional five-pound dumbbell on each knee for the chair position firmer. No weights used for other exercises. If you choose to use the modified pyramid system for thigh work, see pp. 32–33 for review.

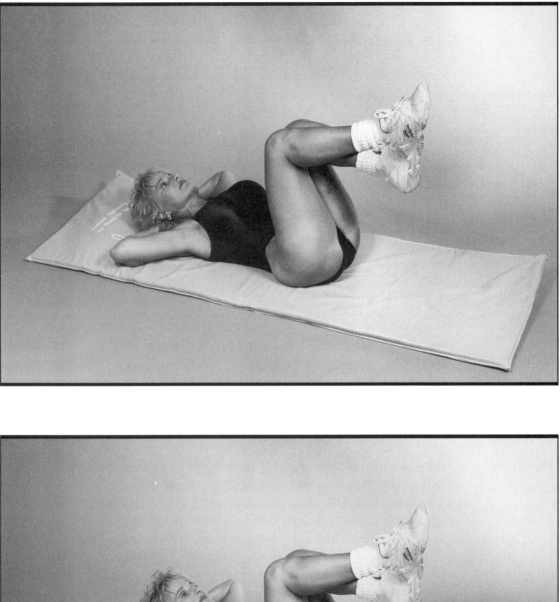

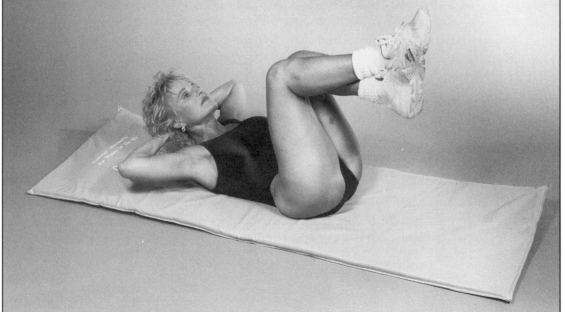

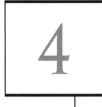

LOWER BUTT SIDE KICK, STRADDLE SQUAT, AND SIDE OBLIQUE CRUNCH

HIPS/BUTTOCKS: LOWER BUTT SIDE KICK SLIMS, FIRMS, SHAPES, AND LIFTS THE ENTIRE LOWER BUTTOCKS AREA.

POSITION Lie on your side with your lower leg bent back on the floor. Your hips should be in line with each other ("stacked"). Support yourself with your lower elbow and place the palm of that hand behind your head. Bring your other arm in front of your chest and place your hand on the floor for support. Bend your leg at the knee and bring it as close to your chest as possible. Flex your toes.

MOVEMENT Keeping your hips in line with each other ("stacked") and leading with your heel, kick your leg out as far as possible and, flexing your buttock as hard as possible, return to the start position. Repeat the movement until you have completed your set. Repeat the set for the other side of your body. Without resting, move to the next exercise in this tri-set, the straddle squat.

TIPS Keep your floor leg bent back in the **L** position and your hips "stacked" throughout the movement for proper support. Be sure to flex your buttocks as hard as possible every time your working leg is extended. Don't hold your breath. Breathe naturally.

MACHINES, ETC. You may substitute this exercise for any exercise done on a rotary butt machine. Set the weight at a comfortable starting weight. Machines vary so you'll have to experiment.

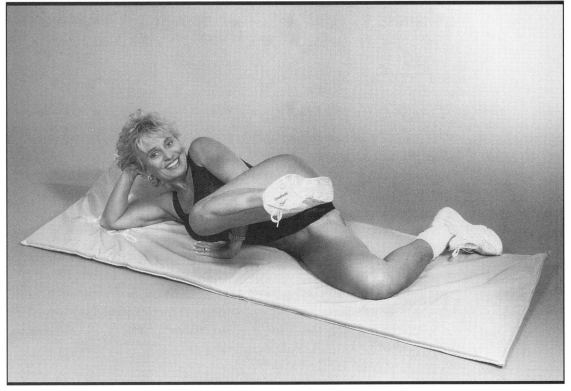

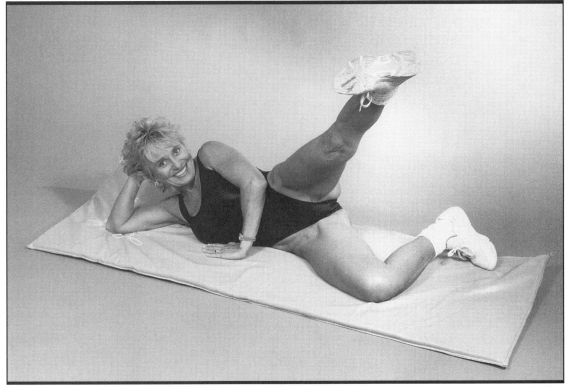

THIGHS: STRADDLE SQUAT DEVELOPS, SHAPES, STRENGTHENS, AND DEFINES THE FRONT THIGH MUSCLE AND HELPS TO TIGHTEN AND TONE THE BUTTOCKS.

POSITION With an optional dumbbell held at each end, palms facing your body, stand with your feet about three to five inches wider than shoulder width apart and your toes pointed slightly outward. Let your arms hang down at your sides. Keep your back erect and your eyes straight ahead.

MOVEMENT Feeling the stretch in your front thigh muscles as you go, descend to an approximate forty-five-degree bend in your knees. Flexing your quadriceps as you go, return to the start position. Willfully flex your quadriceps and repeat the movement until you have completed your set. Without resting, move to the final exercise in this tri-set, the side oblique crunch.

TIPS You may not be able to descend the full distance. Go only as far as possible.

MACHINES, ETC. You may do this exercise with a twenty-pound barbell on your shoulders. You may also do this exercise at any squat machine. Set the weight at a comfortable starting weight. Machines vary, so you'll have to experiment.

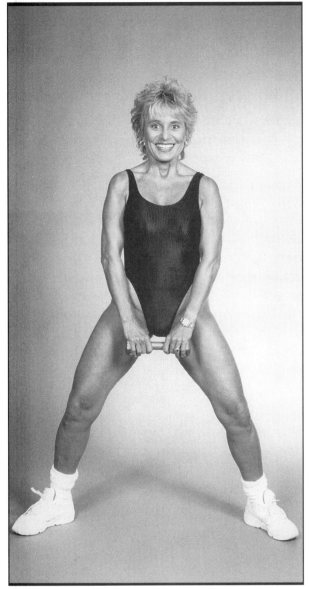

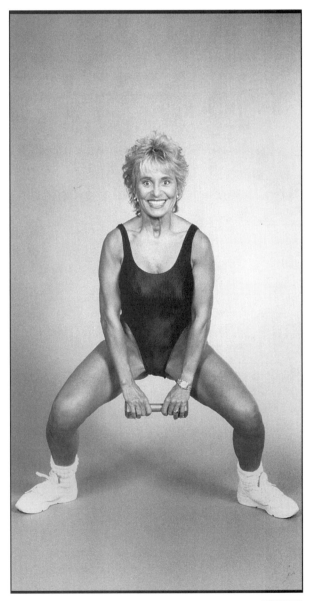

FINISH

ABDOMINALS: SIDE OBLIQUE CRUNCH TIGHTENS, TONES, SHAPES, AND DEFINES THE OBLIQUE MUSCLES.

POSITION   Lie flat on your back with one hand behind your head and your knees bent, the soles of your feet flat on the floor. Extend your other arm down at your side.

MOVEMENT   Supporting your head with your hand, reach toward your ankle with the extended arm, flexing your working oblique muscles as hard as possible as you go. Go as far toward your ankle as possible and return to the start position. Feel the stretch in your working oblique muscles and repeat the movement until you have completed your set. Repeat the set for the other side of your body. Rest an optional fifteen seconds and do another tri-set of this combination. Again, take an optional fifteen-second rest and perform the third and final tri-set of this combination. Rest an optional fifteen seconds and proceed to the first exercise of the next tri-set, the floor feather kick-up.

TIPS   Gently stretch into the hand-to-ankle position. Don't force it. Feel the flex in your oblique muscles as you reach the low position. You may raise your head slightly as you work, supporting your neck with your hand.

MACHINES, ETC.   You may perform this exercise on any rotary torso machine. Set the weight at twenty pounds.

WHAT TO DO:
TRI-SETS,
REPETITIONS,
WEIGHTS
Set 1: Fifteen repetitions each: lower butt side kick, straddle squat, and side oblique crunch. Optional fifteen-second rest.
Set 2: Fifteen repetitions each: lower butt side kick, straddle squat, and side oblique crunch. Optional fifteen-second rest.
Set 3: Fifteen repetitions each: lower butt side kick, straddle squat, and side oblique crunch. Optional fifteen-second rest.

NOTE: Use five-pound dumbbells for straddle squat (optional). No weights required for other exercises. If you choose to use the modified pyramid system for thigh work, see pp. 32–33.

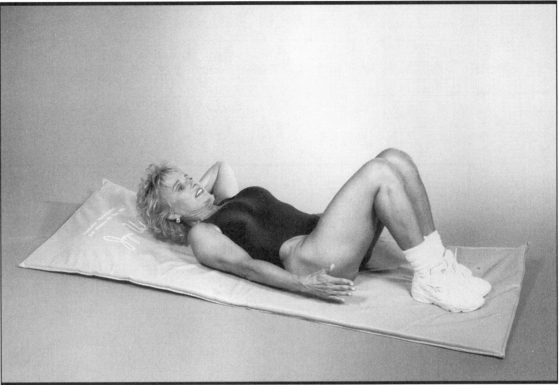

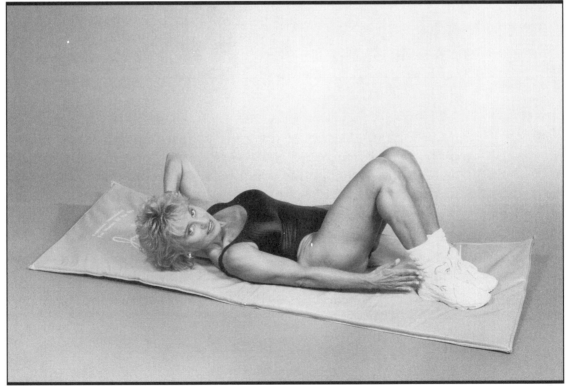

THE BATHING SUIT WORKOUT

5

FLOOR FEATHER KICK-UP, FRONT SQUAT, AND CEILING SEWN LIFT

> **HIPS/BUTTOCKS: FLOOR FEATHER KICK-UP SHAPES, TIGHTENS, TONES, AND LIFTS THE ENTIRE HIPS/BUTTOCKS AREA AND HELPS TO FIRM THE BACK THIGH MUSCLE.**

POSITION   Place yourself in an all-fours position on the floor.

MOVEMENT   Flexing your working foot forward, extend your working leg up and behind you until you cannot go any higher. Your knee should be completely unbent and your extended leg at an approximate ninety-degree angle. In this position, flex your working buttock as hard as possible and, in full control, return to the start position. Repeat the movement until you have completed your set. Repeat the set for the other side of your body. Without resting, move to the next exercise in this tri-set, the front squat.

TIPS   Don't fall into the trap of swinging your leg up and down. Use controlled movements at all times. Flex hard on the up movement and feel the stretch on the down movement. You may perform this exercise by extending your working leg to a parallel-to-the-floor position instead of a ninety-degree angle.

MACHINES, ETC.   You may substitute this exercise for an exercise performed on any hips/buttocks machine. Set the weight at a comfortable starting weight. Machines vary, so you'll have to experiment.

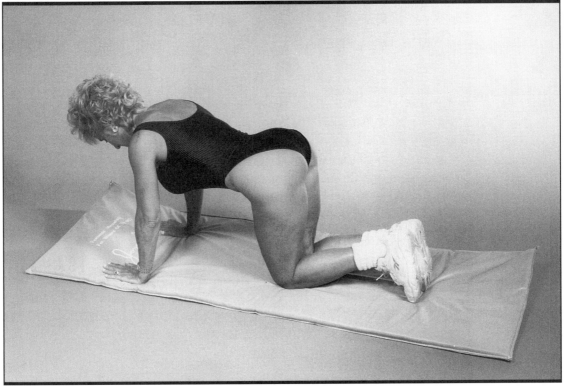

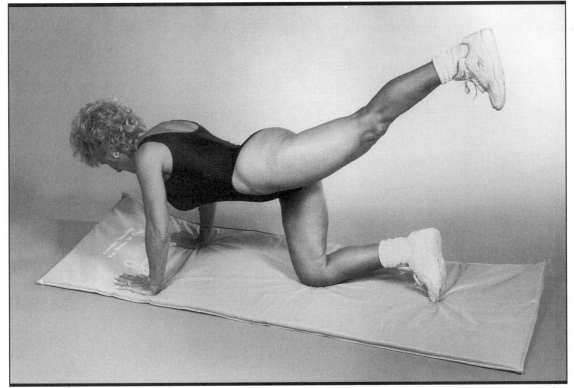

FINISH

THIGHS: FRONT SQUAT DEVELOPS, SHAPES, TONES, AND DEFINES THE FRONT THIGH MUSCLE.

POSITION Stand with your feet a natural width apart and angle your toes out slightly. Hold an optional dumbbell in each hand and cross your arms above your chest. The ends of the dumbbells will be touching your shoulders. Look straight ahead and keep your back straight. Note: If you are not using dumbbells, simply take the position you see in the photo—only without dumbbells.

MOVEMENT Keeping your upper body straight, feel the stretch in your front thighs as you descend to the squat position (descend until your thighs are parallel to the floor or slightly higher). Flex your front thighs as you return to the start position. Give your front thighs an extra-hard flex and repeat the movement until you have completed your set. Without resting, move to the final exercise in this tri-set, the ceiling sewn lift.

TIPS If you find yourself rising up on your toes, try a wider stance!

MACHINES, ETC. You may balance a twenty-five-pound barbell on your chest instead of using the dumbbells. You may substitute the leg press done on any leg-press machine for this or any other squat. Set the machine at a comfortable starting weight. Machines vary, so you'll have to experiment.

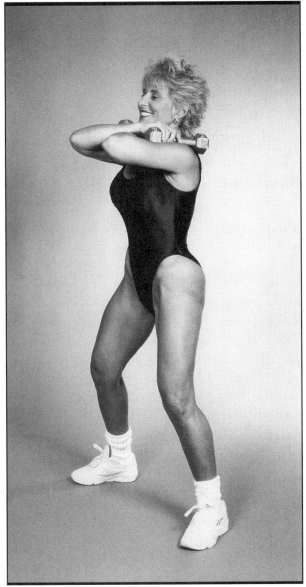

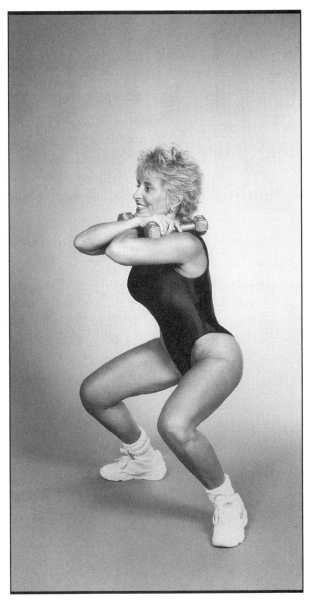

THE BATHING SUIT WORKOUT | **91**

ABDOMINALS: CEILING SEWN LIFT TIGHTENS, TONES, STRENGTHENS, AND DEFINES THE ENTIRE LOWER ABDOMINAL AREA AND HELPS TO STRENGTHEN THE LOWER BACK.

POSITION

Lie on the floor and place your hands behind your head. Raise your legs off the floor, extending your legs fully upward and crossing your legs at the ankles. Push your back into the floor so that there is no "curve" in your back.

MOVEMENT

Making believe that your belly button is sewn to the ground, lift your buttocks off the floor about two to three inches while at the same time flexing your lower abdominal muscles as hard as possible. (Remember, you couldn't go much higher even if you tried. Your belly button is sewn to the ground.) Repeat this movement until you have completed your set. Rest an optional fifteen seconds and do another tri-set of this combination. Again, take an optional fifteen-second rest and perform the third and final tri-set of this combination. Rest an optional fifteen seconds more and proceed to the first exercise of the next tri-set, the lying butt lift.

MACHINES, ETC.

You may substitute this exercise for the leg-raise as demonstrated in my book *Bottoms Up!*

WHAT TO DO:
TRI-SETS,
REPETITIONS,
WEIGHTS

Set 1: Fifteen repetitions each: floor feather kick-up, front squat, ceiling sewn lift. Optional fifteen-second rest.
Set 2: Fifteen repetitions each: floor feather kick-up, front squat, ceiling sewn lift. Optional fifteen-second rest.
Set 3: Fifteen repetitions each: floor feather kick-up, front squat, ceiling sewn lift. Optional fifteen-second rest.

NOTE:

Use five-pound dumbbells for the front squat (optional). No weights required for other exercises. If you choose to use the modified pyramid system for your thighs, see pp. 32–33 for review.

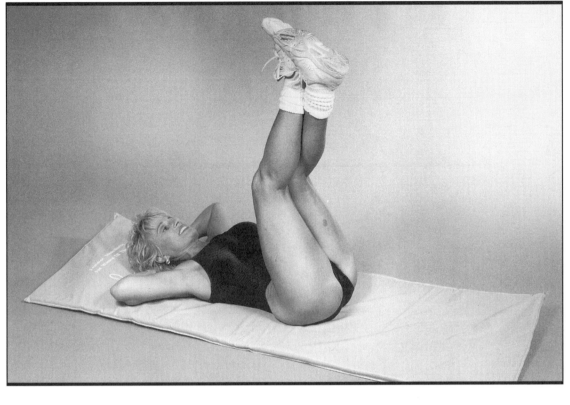

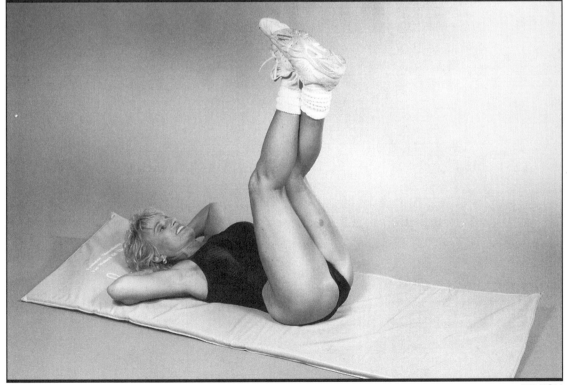

THE BATHING SUIT WORKOUT | **93**

6

LYING BUTT LIFT, LUNGE, AND TOE-REACH CRUNCH

> **HIPS/BUTTOCKS: LYING BUTT LIFT TIGHTENS, TONES, LIFTS, AND SHAPES ENTIRE HIPS/BUTTOCKS AREA.**

POSITION Lie on the floor flat on your back with your knees bent and the soles of your feet flat on the floor. Clasp your hands behind your head, or extend your arms out in front of you and place the palms of your hands on the floor.

MOVEMENT Keeping your back and the soles of your feet flat against the floor and squeezing your entire hips/buttocks area as hard as possible, raise your hips/buttocks off the floor. (You will be raising only about three inches.) On the high position, give your hips/buttocks area an extra-hard flex and return to start. Repeat the movement until you have completed your set. Without resting, move to the next exercise in this tri-set, the lunge.

TIPS Don't be fooled by the small amount of movement in this exercise. If you flex hard on the up movement, it is extremely effective. Don't fall into the trap of getting your back involved in the movement and jerking your entire buttocks off the floor. Maintain intensity by forcing your back and the soles of your feet to remain flat on the floor throughout the movement.

MACHINES, ETC. You may substitute this exercise for any exercise done on a hips/buttocks machine. Set the weight at a comfortable starting weight. Machines vary, so you'll have to experiment.

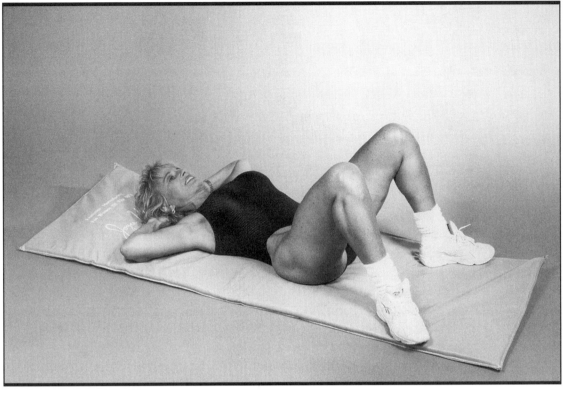

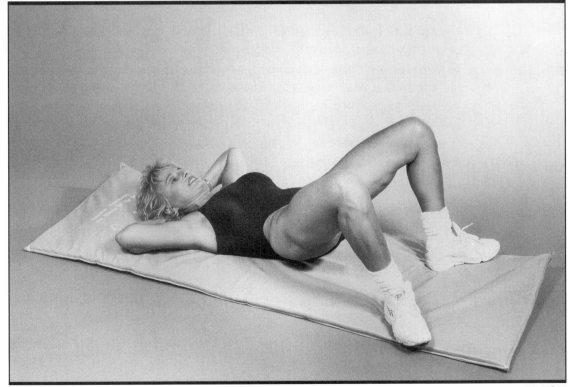

THE BATHING SUIT WORKOUT | 95

THIGHS: LUNGE DEVELOPS, SHAPES, TONES, AND DEFINES THE ENTIRE FRONT THIGH AREA AND HELPS TO LIFT AND SHAPE THE BUTTOCKS.

POSITION

Stand with your feet approximately shoulder width apart, keeping your back straight and looking straight ahead of you. Hold an optional dumbbell in each hand, palms facing your body, with your arms straight down at your sides. (If you are not using weights, simply assume the position in the photograph—without the dumbbells.)

MOVEMENT

Keeping your knee aligned with your toe, bending at the knee, step forward with one foot (about two feet) until you can just about see your toes. (If you cannot see your toes, you have stepped too far.) Feel the flex in your stepping front thigh muscle, and the stretch in your nonstepping front thigh muscle. In full control, return to the start position and give both thighs an extra-hard flex. Repeat the movement for the other leg. Continue this alternate lunging movement until you have completed your set. Without resting, move to the final exercise in this tri-set, the toe-reach crunch.

TIPS

If you're not accustomed to lunges, at first you will be tempted to call yourself uncoordinated, clumsy, and worse. Don't believe it. Ninety-five percent of the people I've worked with stumble about for the first few weeks, then learn balance and love this exercise. Be patient. Everything in time. Don't bounce as you work. Be in full control. As an alternative, you may work one leg at a time, doing one set of lunges for one leg and then the other until all three sets are completed.

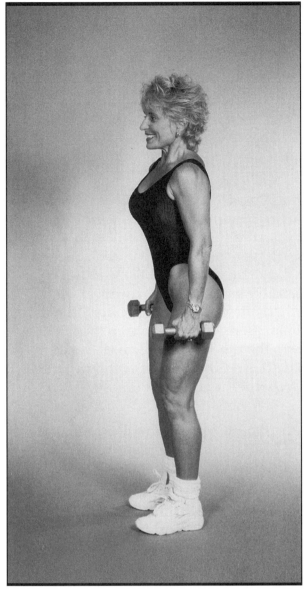

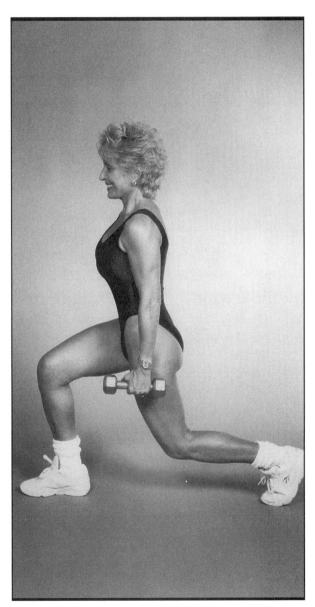

FINISH

ABDOMINALS: TOE-REACH CRUNCH TIGHTENS, TONES, SHAPES, AND DEFINES THE ENTIRE ABDOMINAL AREA.

POSITION

Lie flat on your back on the floor, extending your legs straight up until your knees are only very slightly bent. Extend your arms straight out behind you.

MOVEMENT

Keeping your legs as straight as possible, partially sit up as you extend your arms forward in an attempt to reach for your toes and to touch them with your fingertips (you will not be able to do so), all the while flexing your entire abdominal area. In the highest position, give your abdominal area an extra-hard flex and return to the start position. Without resting, repeat the movement until you have completed your set. Rest an optional fifteen seconds and do another tri-set of this combination. Again, take an optional fifteen-second rest and perform the third and final tri-set of this combination. Rest an optional fifteen seconds more and proceed to the first exercise of the next tri-set, the one-leg prone butt lift.

TIPS

An easier version of this exercise is: Lie with your buttocks against a wall and your legs extended straight up, leaning against the wall. Then perform the movement as described above.

WHAT TO DO: TRI-SETS, REPETITIONS, WEIGHTS

Set 1: Fifteen repetitions each: lying butt lift, lunge, and toe-reach crunch. Optional fifteen-second rest.
Set 2: Fifteen repetitions each: lying butt lift, lunge, and toe-reach crunch. Optional fifteen-second rest.
Set 3: Fifteen repetitions each: lying butt lift, lunge, and toe-reach crunch. Optional fifteen-second rest.

NOTE:

Use five-pound dumbbells for the lunge (optional). No weights are required for other exercises. If you choose to use the modified pyramid system for your thighs, see pp. 32–33 for review.

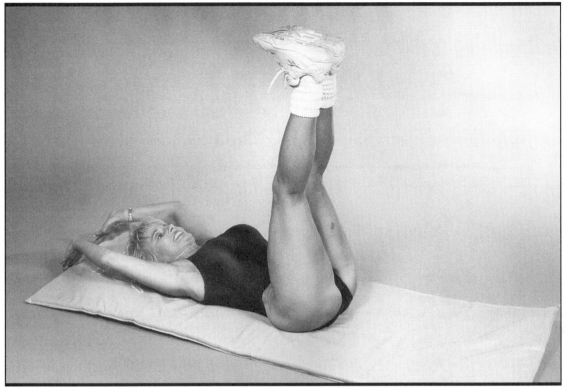

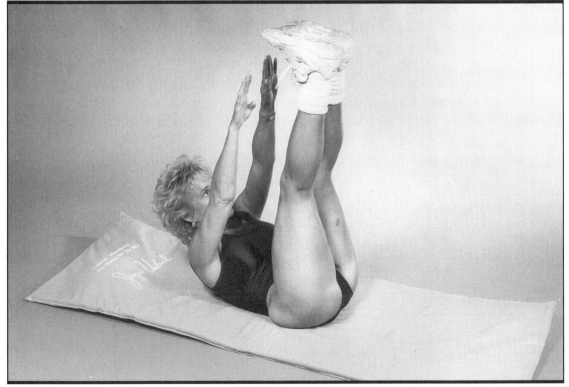

ONE-LEG PRONE BUTT LIFT, REGULAR SQUAT, AND CEILING OBLIQUE REACH

HIPS/BUTTOCKS: ONE-LEG PRONE BUTT LIFT TIGHTENS, TONES, LIFTS, AND SHAPES THE ENTIRE HIPS/BUTTOCKS AREA, AND HELPS TO TONE THE BACK THIGH MUSCLE.

POSITION   Lie on the floor on your stomach, resting your head on the floor or folding your arms and resting your head on your hands. Extend your legs and point your toes, keeping your feet about twelve inches apart.

MOVEMENT   Flexing your hips/buttocks muscles as you go and keeping your knees as locked as possible, lift one leg until you cannot go any higher. Keeping the flex in your working buttock, return to the start position and relax that buttock. Without resting, repeat the movement for the other side of your body. Continue this alternate movement until you have completed your set. Without resting, move to the next exercise in this tri-set, the regular squat.

TIPS   Don't tense your lower back. Relax as you work.

MACHINES, ETC. You may substitute this exercise for any exercise performed on a hips/buttocks machine. Set the weight at a comfortable starting weight. Machines vary, so you'll have to experiment.

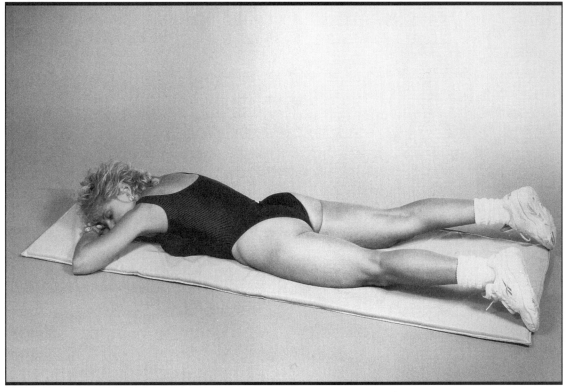

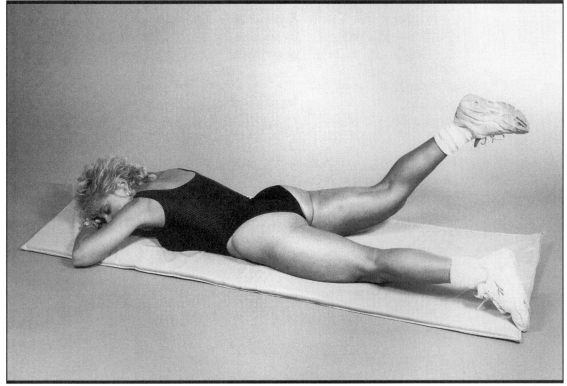

THE BATHING SUIT WORKOUT | **101**

THIGHS: REGULAR SQUAT DEVELOPS, SHAPES, TONES, AND DEFINES THE ENTIRE FRONT THIGH MUSCLE.

POSITION Holding a dumbbell in each hand (optional), palms facing your body, stand with your feet about shoulder width apart and point your toes very slightly outward. Extend your arms down at your sides. Keep your back straight and look straight ahead.

MOVEMENT Feeling the stretch in your front thigh muscles as you go, descend to an approximately forty-five-degree bend in your knees. Flexing your quadriceps as you go, return to the start position. Give your quadriceps an extra-hard flex and repeat the movement until you have completed your set. Without resting, move to the final exercise in this tri-set, the ceiling oblique reach.

TIPS You may not be able to descend the full amount. Go only as far as possible. You may find that you rise on your toes as you descend. If so, adopt a wider stance.

MACHINES, ETC. You may do this exercise with a twenty-pound barbell held on your shoulders. You may also do this exercise at any squat machine. Set the weight at a comfortable starting weight. Machines vary, so you'll have to experiment.

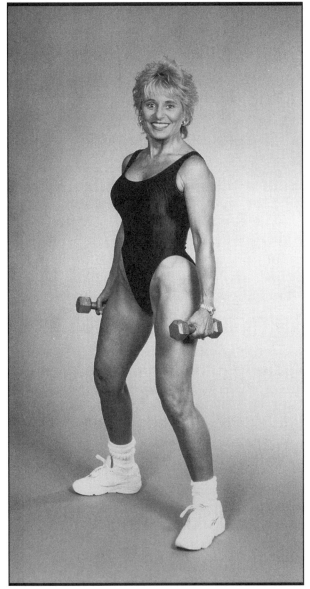

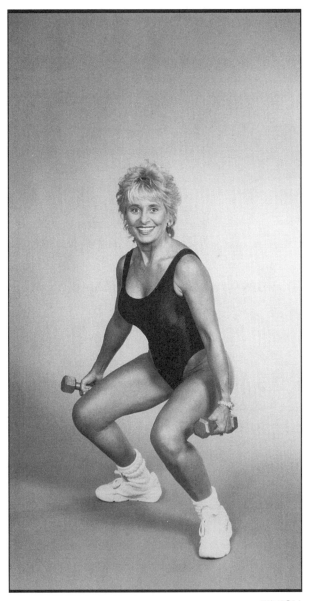

THE BATHING SUIT WORKOUT | **103**

ABDOMINALS: CEILING OBLIQUE REACH TIGHTENS, TONES, DEVELOPS, AND DEFINES THE ENTIRE ABDOMINAL AREA, ESPECIALLY THE OBLIQUE AND UPPER ABDOMINAL MUSCLES.

POSITION

Lie with your back flat on the floor and your legs extended straight up. Place your hands behind your head.

MOVEMENT

Keeping your legs straight up in the air at all times and flexing your working oblique and abdominal muscles as you go, bring your elbow to your opposite knee (or as far as you can go toward the knee). Then extend your arm fully outward. Give your oblique and abdominal muscles an extra-hard flex and, in full control, return to the start position. Without resting, repeat the movement for the other side of your body. Continue this alternating movement until you have completed your set. Rest an optional fifteen seconds and do another tri-set of this combination. Again, take an optional fifteen-second rest and perform the third and final tri-set of this combination. If you are on the regular workout, stop here. Congratulations! You have completed the Bathing Suit Workout. If you are on the Iron, Steel, or Titanium Woman workouts, rest an optional fifteen seconds and proceed to the first exercise of the next tri-set, the standing butt squeeze.

TIPS

Don't fall into the trap of lurching forward as you attempt to touch your elbow to your opposite knee. Maintain control and go only as far as you can go. Beware of the temptation to pull on your head. Use your hands only as *support* for your head.

WHAT TO DO:
TRI-SETS,
REPETITIONS,
WEIGHTS

Set 1: Fifteen repetitions each: one-leg prone butt lift, regular squat, ceiling oblique reach. Optional fifteen-second rest.
Set 2: Fifteen repetitions each: one-leg prone butt lift, regular squat, ceiling oblique reach. Optional fifteen-second rest.
Set 3: Fifteen repetitions each: one-leg prone butt lift, regular squat, ceiling oblique reach. Optional fifteen-second rest.

NOTE:

Use optional five-pound dumbbells for the regular squat. No weights are required for other exercises. If you choose to use the modified pyramid system for your thighs, see pp. 32–33 for review.

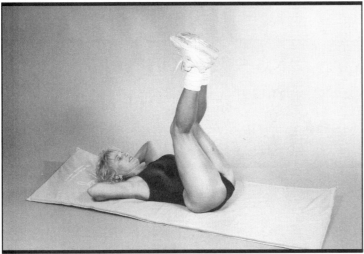

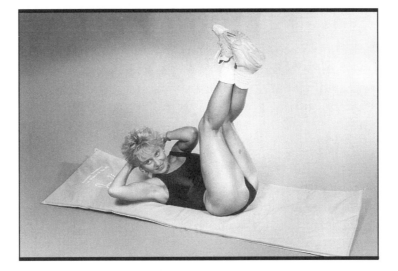

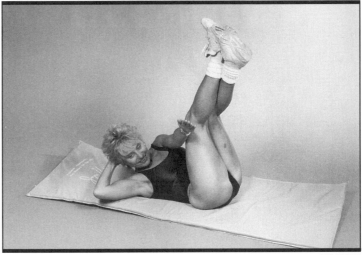

FINISH

8

STANDING BUTT SQUEEZE, HACK SQUAT, AND KNEE-IN

(FOR IRON WOMAN, STEEL WOMAN, AND TITANIUM WOMAN WORKOUTS)

HIPS/BUTTOCKS: STANDING BUTT SQUEEZE TIGHTENS, TONES, LIFTS, AND SHAPES THE ENTIRE HIPS/BUTTOCKS AREA.

POSITION   Holding an optional dumbbell in each hand, palms facing your body and arms straight at your side, stand with your feet a natural width apart with your back straight. Bend at the knees slightly, so that your body is about four inches lower to the ground.

MOVEMENT   Flexing your entire hips/buttocks area as hard as possible, slowly rise to a full standing position. When you reach the highest point, give your hips/buttocks area an extra-hard flex. Repeat the movement until you have completed your set. Without resting, move to the next exercise in this tri-set, the hack squat.

TIPS   Don't do this in front of the opposite sex! I won't be responsible.

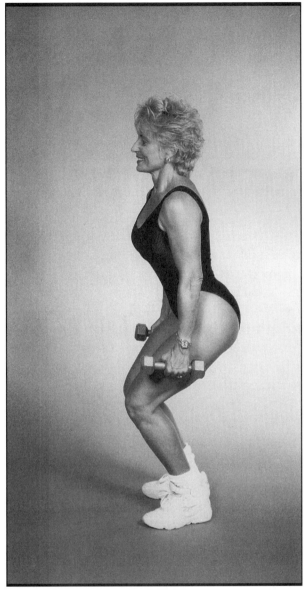

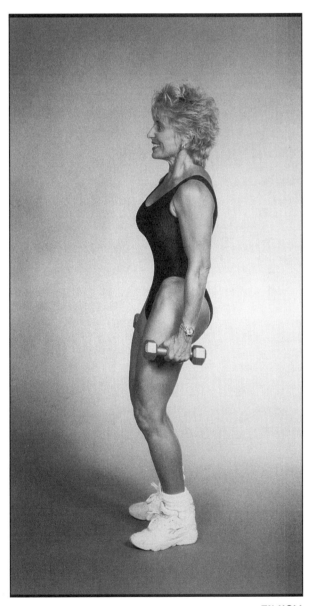

THE BATHING SUIT WORKOUT | 107

THIGHS: HACK SQUAT TIGHTENS, TONES, STRENGTHENS, AND DEFINES THE ENTIRE FRONT THIGH MUSCLE AND HELPS TO DEVELOP AND TONE THE BACK THIGH MUSCLE AND TO REMOVE SADDLEBAGS.

POSITION Stand with your feet a natural width apart. Hold an optional dumbbell in each hand, behind your back and in line with each buttock and back thigh. Your palms will be facing away from your body.

MOVEMENT Keeping the dumbbells in position as you go, bend at the knee until you are in a full squat or as far as your knees will allow. Feel the stretch in your front thigh muscles. Flexing your front thigh muscles as you go and keeping the dumbbells in line with your buttocks and back thighs, return to the start position. Give your front thighs an extra-hard flex and repeat the movement until you have completed your set. Without resting, move to the third and final exercise in this tri-set, the knee-in.

TIPS If you rise up on your toes, take a wider stance.

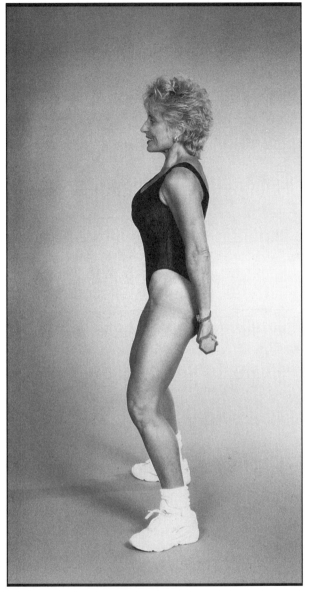

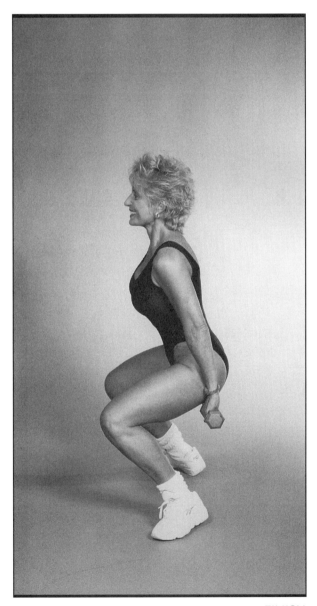

THE BATHING SUIT WORKOUT | 109

ABDOMINALS: KNEE-IN TIGHTENS, TONES, STRENGTHENS, AND DEFINES THE ENTIRE LOWER ABDOMINAL AREA.

POSITION   Lie flat on your back on the floor and extend your legs out in front of you with your knees very slightly bent.

MOVEMENT   Flexing your lower abdominal muscles as you go and keeping your knees together and your back flat on the floor, pull your knees toward your chest until you cannot go any farther. Keeping the tension on your lower abdominal muscles, return to the start position and repeat the movement until you have completed your set. Rest an optional fifteen seconds and do another tri-set of this combination. Again, take an optional fifteen-second rest and perform the third and final tri-set of this combination. If you are on the Iron Woman workout, stop here. Congratulations! You have completed your Bathing Suit Workout. If you are on the Steel Woman workout or the Titanium Woman workout, rest an optional fifteen seconds and proceed to the first exercise of the next tri-set, the reverse-lunge lift.

TIPS   Don't jerk your knees toward your chest. Use controlled movements, and remember to keep the pressure on your abdominals throughout the movement.

WHAT TO DO:
TRI-SETS,
REPETITIONS,
WEIGHTS

Set 1: Fifteen repetitions each: standing butt squeeze, hack squat, knee-in. Optional fifteen-second rest.
Set 2: Fifteen repetitions each: standing butt squeeze, hack squat, knee-in. Optional fifteen-second rest.
Set 3: Fifteen repetitions each: standing butt squeeze, hack squat, knee-in. Optional fifteen-second rest.

NOTE: Hold five-pound dumbbells in each hand for the standing butt squeeze as for an anchor (optional), and use five-pound dumbbells for the hack squat (also optional). No weights are required for other exercises. If you choose to use the modified pyramid system for thighs, see pp. 32–33 for review. There is no need to pyramid when doing butt work. The weights are used only as an anchor.

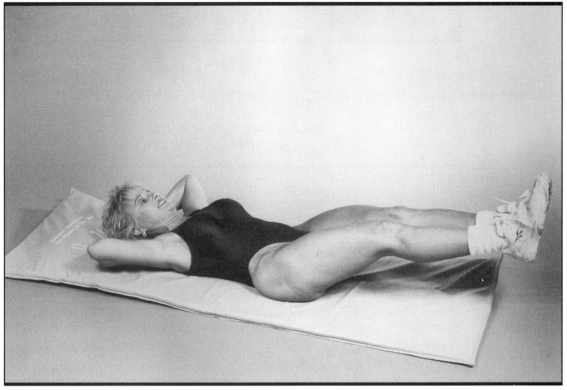

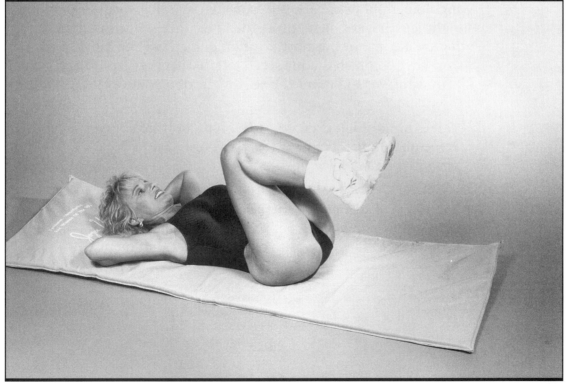

9

REVERSE-LUNGE LIFT, BENT-KNEE DEADLIFT, AND SIT-UP

(FOR STEEL WOMAN AND TITANIUM WOMAN WORKOUTS)

HIPS/BUTTOCKS: REVERSE-LUNGE LIFT TIGHTENS, TONES, SHAPES, AND LIFTS THE ENTIRE HIPS/BUTTOCKS AREA.

POSITION   Stand with your left leg forward, bent at the knee, and your right leg nearly straight and about two feet behind your left leg. Extend your left arm back and your right arm forward. (You will be in a lunge position.)

MOVEMENT   Keeping your left leg in place, bending your right knee, and swinging your right arm back and your left arm forward, move your right leg forward, bending at the knee until you cannot go any higher. Return to the start position and repeat the movement until you have completed your set. (Note: Whichever leg is back, that arm is forward!) Repeat the set for the other side of your body.

TIPS   This is not a thigh exercise—it's a hips/buttocks exercise. Remember to flex your buttocks as hard as possible each time you reach the straight-leg position.

MACHINES, ETC. You may substitute this exercise for any exercise done on a hips/buttocks machine. Set the weight at a comfortable starting weight. Machines vary, so you'll have to experiment.

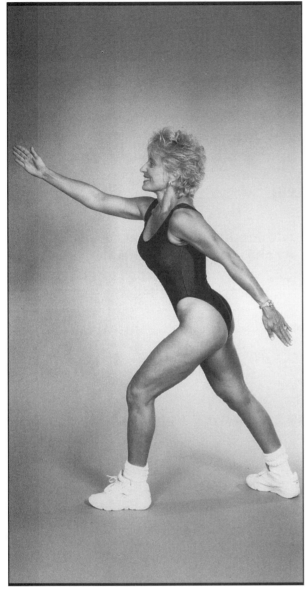

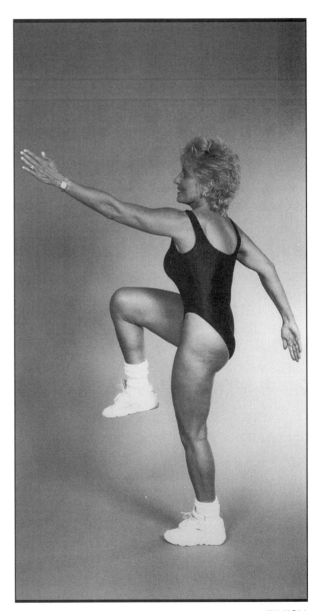

THE BATHING SUIT WORKOUT | 113

THIGHS: BENT-KNEE DEADLIFT TIGHTENS, TONES, STRENGTHENS, AND SHAPES THE BACK THIGH AREA AND HELPS TO STRENGTHEN THE BACK.

POSITION   With an optional dumbbell in each hand, palms facing your body, stand with your feet a natural width apart and bend at the knees while holding a dumbbell in front of each knee. If you are not using weights, simply assume the position you see in the photograph—only without dumbbells.

MOVEMENT   Flexing your back thigh and buttocks muscles as you go, rise to a standing position and squeeze your butt and back thigh muscles as hard as possible. Without resting, repeat the movement until you have completed your set. Without resting, move the final exercise in this tri-set, the sit-up.

TIPS   The effectiveness of this exercise depends upon strict performance and intense flexing.

MACHINES, ETC.   You may perform this exercise with a twenty-pound barbell.

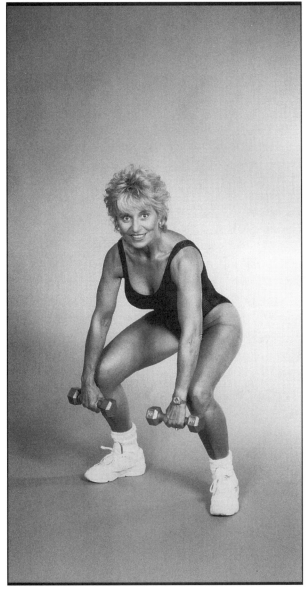

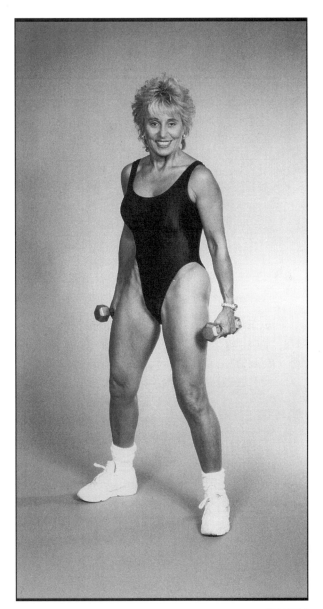

FINISH

ABDOMINALS: SIT-UP TIGHTENS, TONES, STRENGTHENS, AND DEFINES THE UPPER ABDOMINAL AREA.

POSITION

Lie flat on your back on the floor and bend your knees so that the soles of your feet are touching the floor. Place your hands behind your head or cross them in front of you on your stomach or chest.

MOVEMENT

Flexing your upper abdominals as you go, raise yourself off the floor until you are in a nearly perpendicular position. In full control, lower yourself to the start position and repeat the movement until you have completed your set. Rest an optional fifteen seconds and do another tri-set of this combination. Again, take an optional fifteen-second rest and perform your third and final tri-set of this combination. If you are on the Steel Woman workout, stop here. Congratulations! You have completed your Bathing Suit Workout. If you are on the Titanium Woman workout, rest an optional fifteen seconds more and proceed to the first exercise of the next tri-set, the straight leg kick-up.

TIPS

Don't jerk up, but rather curl to the up position. If necessary, you may cross your ankles for leverage, or place your ankles under a piece of furniture.

WHAT TO DO:
TRI-SETS,
REPETITIONS,
WEIGHTS

Set 1: Fifteen repetitions each: reverse-lunge lift, bent-knee deadlift, sit-up. Optional fifteen-second rest.
Set 2: Fifteen repetitions each: reverse-lunge lift, bent-knee deadlift, sit-up. Optional fifteen-second rest.
Set 3: Fifteen repetitions each: reverse-lunge lift, bent-knee deadlift, sit-up. Optional fifteen-second rest.

NOTE:

Use five-pound dumbbells for the bent-knee deadlift (optional). No weights are used for other exercises. If you choose to use the modified pyramid system for your thighs, see pp. 32–33 for review.

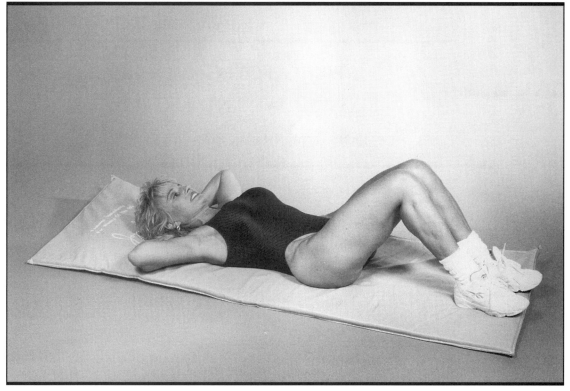

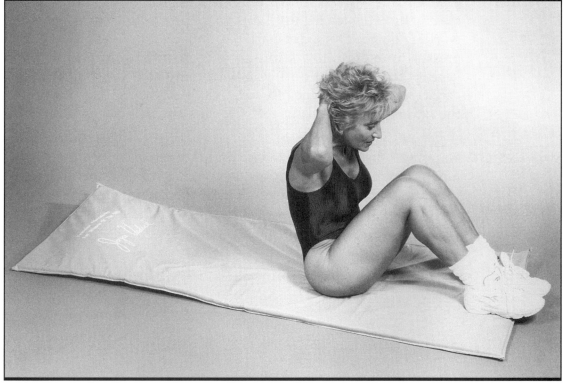

THE BATHING SUIT WORKOUT | 117

10

STRAIGHT-LEG KICK-UP, SISSY SQUAT, AND LEG RAISE

(FOR TITANIUM WOMAN WORKOUT)

> **HIPS/BUTTOCKS, STRAIGHT-LEG KICK-UP TIGHTENS, TONES, LIFTS, AND SHAPES THE ENTIRE BUTTOCKS AREA AND HELPS TO REMOVE "SADDLEBAGS."**

POSITION — Take an all-fours position on the floor. Extend one leg straight out behind you, in line with your body, and flex the foot of that leg forward.

MOVEMENT — Flexing your working buttock as hard as possible as you move, raise your extended leg until it is parallel to your body. Give your working buttock an extra-hard flex and, continuing to keep the pressure on your buttock muscle, return to the start position. Repeat the movement until you have completed your set. Repeat the set for the other side of your body. Without resting, move to the next exercise in this tri-set, the sissy squat.

MACHINES, ETC. — You may substitute this exercise for any exercise done on a hips/buttocks machine. Set the weight at a comfortable starting weight. Machines vary, so you'll have to experiment. You may perform a variation of this exercise with your toes pointed back and by raising your leg as high as possible.

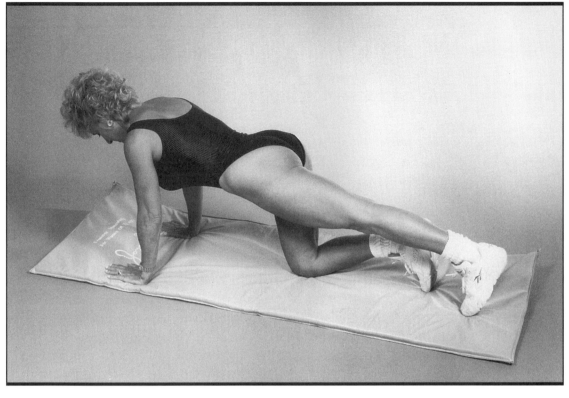

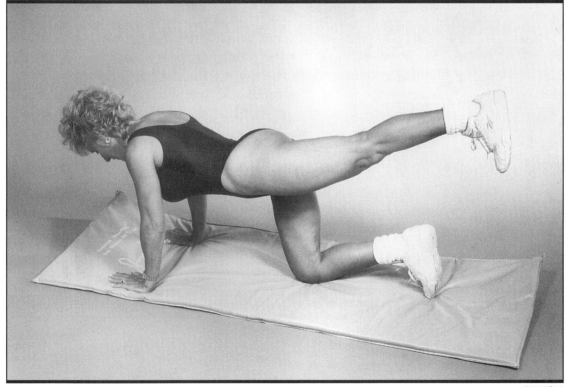

THIGH: SISSY SQUAT TIGHTENS, TONES, STRENGTHENS, AND DEFINES THE FRONT THIGH MUSCLE, GIVES DEFINITION TO THE INNER THIGH, HELPS TO LIFT THE BUTTOCKS AND TONE THE BACK THIGH MUSCLE.

POSITION

Stand with your feet about five inches apart and your toes pointed slightly outward. Place one hand on a stable object for support. Note: Even if you are taking advantage of the optional weights, no weights are used with this thigh exercise.

MOVEMENT

Applying tension to your front, inner, and back thigh muscles as you go, raise yourself on your toes. At the same time, lean your upper body back as far as you can go and squeeze your buttocks as hard as possible. You will be completely up on your toes at this point and you will feel an extreme stretch in your front thigh muscles. Be sure that your hips are in line with your ankles as you work. Continuing to keep the pressure on your thigh and buttocks muscles, return to the start position and repeat the movement until you have completed your set. Without resting, move to the final exercise in this tri-set, the leg raise.

TIPS

At first this exercise will seem awkward, especially if you try to follow the words and not the photographs. Look at the picture and imitate what I do. In time you'll appreciate this weightless exercise for its ability to stretch and define your front thighs fully. Advanced bodybuilders perform this exercise with a weight-belt attached to their waists.

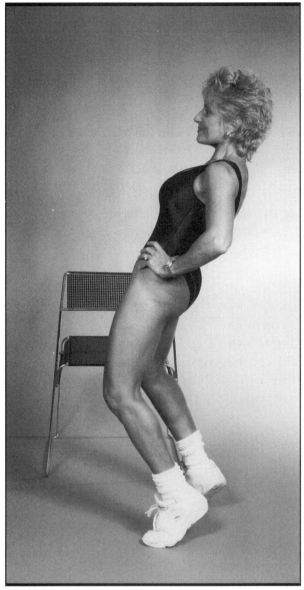

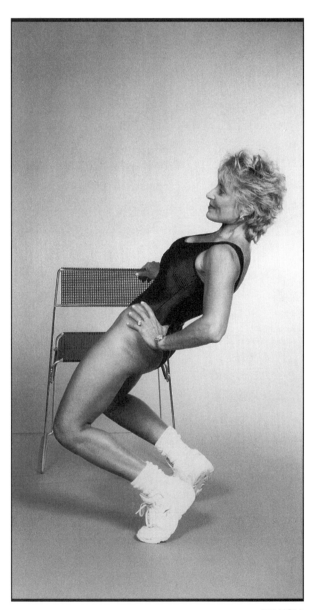

THE BATHING SUIT WORKOUT | 121

ABDOMINALS: LEG RAISE TIGHTENS, TONES, STRENGTHENS, AND DEFINES THE LOWER ABDOMINAL AREA.

POSITION   Lie flat on your back and place your hands behind your head or at the sides of a bench. Bend at the knees and keep your shoulders and back grounded as you work.

MOVEMENT   Flexing your lower abdominal muscles as you go and, keeping your knees moderately bent, raise your legs until they are perpendicular to the floor. Give your lower abdominals an extra-hard flex and, in full control, return to the start position—but do not touch the ground with your feet. Without resting, repeat the movement until you have completed your set. Rest an optional fifteen seconds and do another tri-set of this combination. Again, take an optional fifteen-second rest and perform the third and final tri-set of this combination. Congratulations! You have completed the Bathing Suit Titanium Woman workout.

TIPS   Don't arch your back as you work. Keep it flat on the floor. Be sure to keep your knees and ankles together throughout the movement.

MACHINES, ETC.   You may perform this exercise on any Roman chair by extending your legs until they are parallel to the floor.

WHAT TO DO:
TRI-SETS,
REPETITIONS,
WEIGHTS
Set 1: Fifteen repetitions each: straight-leg kick-up, sissy squat, leg raise. Optional fifteen-second rest.
Set 2: Fifteen repetitions each: straight-leg kick-up, sissy squat, leg raise. Optional fifteen-second rest.
Set 3: Fifteen repetitions each: straight-leg kick-up, sissy squat, leg raise. Optional fifteen-second rest.

NOTE: No weights are used for any exercise in this tri-set, not even thighs!

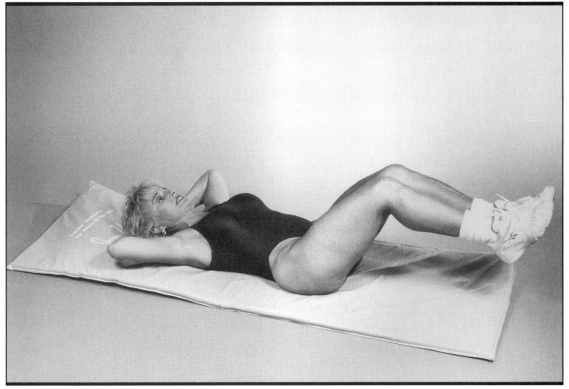

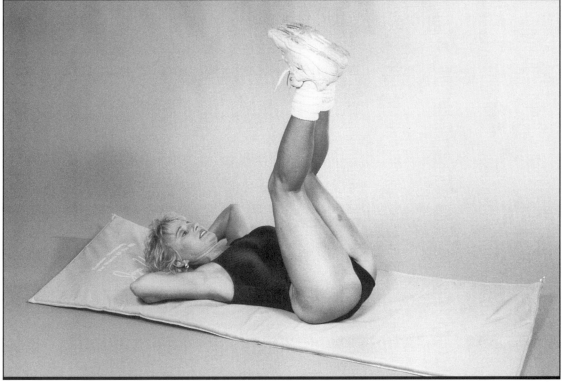

Review of Exercises Found in This Workout

HIPS/BUTTOCKS	THIGHS	ABDOMINALS
1. Saddlebag stripper	Lying inner thigh lift	Knee-raised oblique crunch
2. Lower butt curl	Leg curl	Bent-knee sewn lift
3. Lower butt crunch	Chair position firmer	Knee-raised crunch
4. Lower butt side kick	Straddle squat	Side oblique crunch
5. Floor feather kick-up	Front squat	Ceiling sewn lift
6. Lying butt lift	Lunge	Toe-reach crunch
7. One-leg prone butt lift	Regular squat	Ceiling oblique reach
8. Standing butt squeeze (Iron, Steel, and Titanium Woman workouts)	Hack squat	Knee-in
9. Reverse-lunge lift (Steel and Titanium Woman workouts)	Bent-knee deadlift	Sit-up
10. Straight-leg knee-up (Titanium Woman workout)	Sissy squat	Leg raise

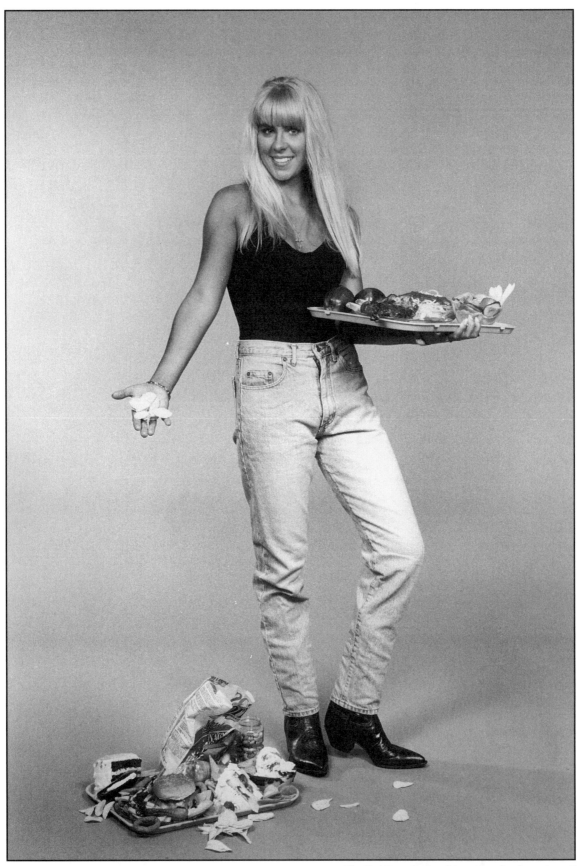

Marthe, Joyce's daughter, who also loves to eat!

7

THE
BATHING SUIT DIET

You know what to do for exercise; now you must learn about the other half of your fitness program: what to eat! Diet (meaning what you eat on a daily basis) is the key to showing off your hard-earned hard body! Without the diet, your fat would cover the muscles. You would feel firmer, but you wouldn't look sleek and shapely.

But what about if you're not overweight to begin with—in fact, you may even be a bit too thin—but your body is soft and mushy? Do you have to follow this eating plan? No. You can continue to eat your regular fare—assuming it is a healthy diet. You and your doctor can decide upon that. For the rest of us poor souls, we must follow the diet and thank God that we have the knowledge that will allow us to eat plenty of food and still lose our excess body fat.

A Balanced, Low-Fat—Not Nonfat—Diet is the Key

As mentioned in Chapter 2, the three macronutrients, carbohydrates, protein, and fats, are needed by the body in a certain balance in order to maintain good health and to keep the body lean and fit. We've already gone into details about fat, which is needed in a lower percentage by the body than the carbohydrates, and in about an equal percentage to protein. In this chapter you'll learn the details about protein and carbohydrate, and how to balance them along with fat in your diet so that day by day you will lose your excess body fat. The percentages of the three food elements you will eat are not exact, but to round it off, you'll be consuming about 15 percent fat, 15 percent protein, and 70 percent carbohydrates.

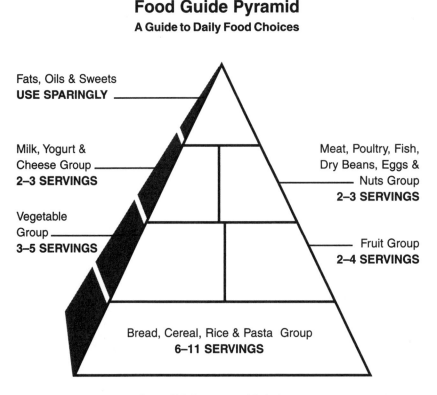

Food Guide Pyramid
A Guide to Daily Food Choices

Fats, Oils & Sweets
USE SPARINGLY

Milk, Yogurt &
Cheese Group
2–3 SERVINGS

Meat, Poultry, Fish,
Dry Beans, Eggs &
Nuts Group
2–3 SERVINGS

Vegetable
Group
3–5 SERVINGS

Fruit Group
2–4 SERVINGS

Bread, Cereal, Rice & Pasta Group
6–11 SERVINGS

Source: U.S. Department of Agriculture

The USDA has come out with a "food pyramid" that outlines what is considered by health and nutrition experts to be a balanced diet. Here it is:

The bare minimum of fats and refined simple carbohydrates

2–3 servings of protein

6–11 servings starches (breads, grains, rice, pasta, cereal)

3–5 servings of vegetables (unlimited complex carbohydrates)

2–4 fruits

1–2 servings of dairy products

I have based the diet plan in this chapter on the food pyramid. However, I've changed the maximum number of the "starches" group to ten servings. I've also renamed that category and called it "limited complex carbohydrates." In addition, I must advise you that if you want to lose your excess body fat at the quickest possible pace, except for "unlimited complex carbohydrates" keep to the lower end of the food allowances. ("Unlimited complex carbohydrates" work in reverse. The more you eat of them, the faster you will lose your excess body fat. You'll understand why as you read this chapter.) Finally, I've given you food lists from which to choose your food portions, in order to insure that your diet remains low-fat and at the same time nutritious.

Protein

If you read Chapter 2, you already know that you are not allowed to eat pure fat in any form (butter, margarine, etc.). You must rely on the other two food sources to get your fat! Protein will be your main source of fat, specifically, low-fat sources of protein.

Only about 15 percent of your food intake will be protein. You will get your 15 percent protein simply by eating two to three portions (listed below) of protein per day. You don't have to calculate anything. I've done it for you.

Protein has a strange characteristic. It can only be used productively by your body in small amounts at a time. If you eat it in large portions, it ends up getting stored on your body as fat. (Note: For some people, 15 percent of protein is too much. If you feel this way, you can increase your carbohydrate intake and lower your protein intake. Simply reduce the portions of protein to four ounces and have only two portions instead of three.)

Protein is considered to be the "building block" of the body because it is responsible for the major content of muscle, skin, hair, nails, blood, and internal organs. It is also responsible for body repair, water balance, and hormone production that controls metabolism, growth, and sexual development, and regulates the acid–alkaline balance of the blood and tissues.

In other books, I've stated that the ideal amount of protein consumption if you work out with weights is about 1/2 gram of protein per day for each pound of body weight. (Bodybuilders often consume double that amount.) For example, if you weigh 120 pounds, you could consume sixty grams of protein in a day. I stand by that figure here; however, I will modify it to say that you could consume much less if you wish. The bare minimum would be forty-four grams a day for women.

But where will you get your protein? There are approximately five grams of protein per ounce of poultry, and six grams per ounce of fish. So if you wish to consume the smaller portion of four ounces of fish instead of six ounces, you will have had twenty-four grams of protein in a serving. Later in the day you might consume four ounces of chicken—twenty grams of protein. That adds up to forty-four grams of protein. You're allowed another portion of protein (you are allowed two to three portions a day) but if you don't feel like having any more protein, that's okay. You have consumed your minimum required amount for good health.

Low-Fat Sources of Protein

All poultry is without skin and cooked without fat! I'm listing the fat grams for your convenience.

Poultry (4 oz. cooked)	Grams of Fat	Grams of Protein
Turkey breast	1	34
Turkey drumstick	4.5	33
Turkey thigh	5	31
Chicken breast	4.5	35
Chicken drumstick	6.8	37
Chicken thigh	5	31

Fish (4 oz.)	Grams of Fat	Grams of Protein
Mahi-mahi (dolphin fish)	0.8	20.8
Haddock	1	23
Cod	1	26
Abalone	1	16
Sole	1	19
Pike	1	25
Scallops	1	26
Tuna in water	1	34
Squid	1.8	20
Flounder	2.3	34
Red snapper	2.3	26
Sea bass	3.4	25
Halibut	4	31
Trout	4	30

Other Sources of Protein

Food Product	Grams of Fat	Grams of Protein
4 ounces low-fat yogurt	2	6
4 ounces nonfat yogurt	0	7
8 ounces 1 percent milk	3	8
8 ounces skim milk	1	8
4 ounces (1/2 cup) 1% cottage cheese	1	14
4 ounces (1/2 cup) full-fat cottage cheese	5	14
3 egg whites	2	9
1/2 cup beans	1	9
1/2 cup soft tofu	6	10
1/2 cup firm tofu	11	19

YOU WILL GET MUCH OF YOUR FAT ALLOTMENT FROM PROTEIN

You will notice that I've included the fat grams in the above calculations. That is because you will get a major part of your 15 percent or twenty to twenty-five grams of fat from your protein allotment. The rest will come from limited complex carbohydrates (sometimes called starches). You don't have to count the traces of fat found in unlimited complex carbohydrates and fresh fruit.

Carbohydrates

Most of your food intake (70 percent) should come from carbohydrates—they are the energy food for both body and mind. If you deprive your body of them, you feel enervated and irritable!

Carbohydrates are divided into two categories. The first is simple carbohydrates or sugars, which itself divides into two categories: refined (sugars found in candy, cake, doughnuts, white flour, etc.) and unrefined (sugars found in fruit). The second category is complex carbohydrates, which consist of vegetables, grains, and fiber.

You get an immediate shot of energy from simple carbohydrates. Complex carbohydrates, on the other hand, supply gradually released energy. The majority of your carbohydrate consumption will come from the latter group. We'll discuss the carbohydrates in order, from most consumed to least consumed in the ideal diet.

COMPLEX CARBOHYDRATES: YOUR MAIN FOOD SOURCE

As mentioned above, complex carbohydrates include all vegetables, grains, and fiber. But there are two types of complex carbohydrates: low caloric density and high caloric density. (Caloric density is the number of calories per weight of a particular food.) It is better to eat foods low in caloric density—foods that weigh more but have fewer calories—than foods in high caloric density—foods that weigh less and have more calories. Why?

If you're anything like me, you like to eat until you feel full. Since your calories are limited, you can't eat enough of the lighter-weight foods and still feel satisfied. Since your stomach can only hold about two pounds of food, it's better to eat two pounds of vegetables than two pounds of bread, even if that bread is whole-wheat bread. The bread would cost you too many calories.

Complex carbohydrates that are low in caloric density include all vegetables, pasta, rice, and hot cereals. Of course this doesn't mean you must eliminate healthful low-caloric-density foods such as wheat bread, cold cereals, rice cakes, etc. It just means that, if you want to feel full without eating too much, you're better off filling up on the high-caloric-density foods.

BEWARE: SOME CARBOHYDRATES CAN HINDER FAT BURNING

Processed carbohydrates, such as all forms of sugar and white breads, rice, and pasta can hinder fat burning. Why? When such foods are consumed, large amounts of glucose are released to the bloodstream, causing your body to produce high levels of insulin, which in turn inhibits hormone-sensitive lipase—the enzyme that is responsible for draining fat from the cells! A simple rule of thumb is: sugar very rarely, and brown is better than white!

6–10 SERVINGS OF LIMITED COMPLEX CARBOHYDRATES (STARCHES)

This group of complex carbohydrates includes bread, cereal, rice, pasta, and all grains, plus two high-starch vegetables.

One Serving Equals	Fat Grams
1 slice whole-wheat bread	.5
1/2 bagel	.6
1/2 English or bran muffin	.6
1/2 cup cooked hot cereal	1

One Serving Equals	Fat Grams
1 cup dry cold cereal	1
1/2 cup cooked pasta or rice	.5
1 ounce pretzels	0–1
4 low-fat medium-sized crackers or 2 rice cakes	.6
1 large potato or 1 medium-sized yam or sweet potato	.1
1 cup corn or 1 large corn on the cob	.9

You will have a minimum of six servings and a maximum of ten servings for the day—and still lose weight. The less weight you have to lose, the closer you will have to go to the minimum number!

3–12 OR MORE SERVINGS OF VEGETABLES: UNLIMITED COMPLEX CARBOHYDRATES

You can and should eat as much as you please of these vegetables. In fact, it is mandatory for good health that you have at least three servings per day. However, for our purposes, three servings is not enough. If you keep to the bare minimum, you will probably feel hungry all the time. Why? Your other foods are very limited. Once you use up your allotment of those foods, you'll have two choices. Either feel hungry or eat vegetables!

1 Serving of Unlimited Complex Carbohydrates Equals:

1/2 cup cooked or 1 cup raw equals a serving.

Asparagus	Leeks
Broccoli	Lettuce
Brussels sprouts	Mushrooms
Cabbage, Chinese cabbage	Okra
Carrots	Onions
Cauliflower	Peppers, green or red
Celery	Radishes
Chicory	Rutabagas
Collard greens	Shallots
Cucumber	Sprouts
Eggplant	Squash (summer or zucchini)
Endive	Tomatoes
Escarole	Turnips
Kale	

Note: One tomato, cucumber, or pepper counts as a serving. As mentioned above, you don't have to count the fat grams in the unlimited vegetables or fruits.

SIMPLE CARBOHYDRATES: FRUIT

Both fruit and fruit juice are simple unrefined carbohydrates (sugars), but fruit is much better for you than juice because, as mentioned in Chapter 2, fruit juices function as do pure sugar or refined carbohydrates: They cause your insulin level to rise, which in turn can cause hunger and hinder fat burning. In addition, when you drink juice instead of eating the real fruit, you deprive yourself of the nutritious fiber and bulk of the fruit—and the opportunity to feel full!

2–4 SIMPLE CARBOHYDRATES (FRUIT) PER DAY

One Serving of Fruit Equals:
One medium to large piece of any fruit: apple, orange, pear, banana, etc.
1 cup berries of any kind or papaya
1 1/2 cups strawberries, watermelon
1/2 cantaloupe, grapefruit, large plantain
15 cherries
20 grapes
3 persimmons, kumquats,
fresh prunes
*1/2 cup juice
1/4 honeydew or pineapple
2 plums or tangerines
1 serving of nonfat cake, cookies, candy, jam, jelly, etc. (You will have this no more than twice a week. A serving is whatever is designated on the package as a serving.)

*Note: It is always better to have fruit rather than fruit juce. Fruit adds fiber to your diet and fills up your stomach. Juice may trigger a hunger response.

SIMPLE REFINED CARBOHYDRATES

Since simple refined carbohydrates can hinder your fat-burning process and must be kept to a minimum in your diet. So, except for a small amount, leave them out of your diet. However, when you do indulge, you will of course choose the low-fat, or better, the nonfat variety. As noted in your fruit food list, you can have a simple refined carbohydrate in place of a fruit. Later, you will be given an opportunity to have a simple refined carbohydrate in place of a dairy product (like nonfat sugar-containing ice cream).

WHAT ABOUT DAIRY?

2–3 DAIRY FOODS PER DAY

One Serving Equals:

1 glass of skim or 1 percent milk

8 oz. nonfat or 1 percent yogurt

4 oz. nonfat or 1 percent cottage cheese

2 tbsp. nonfat cream cheese

11/2 slices (ounces) nonfat cheese

1/2 cup nonfat ice cream, no more than twice a week

WHAT ABOUT FIBER AND WHERE IS IT FOUND?

Fiber is found in vegetables and fruit. Your daily fiber intake should be at least thirty grams, but you won't have to count fiber grams because if you follow this eating plan, you'll automatically get more than your bare minimum!

Fiber helps to prevent all kinds of diseases, helps to move fat out of your system, and helps you to eliminate foods (through bowel movement).

WHY IS FIBER GOOD FOR YOUR HEALTH?

There are two types of fiber. First, there is **soluble fiber**, which is found in oat bran, psyllium, fresh fruits and vegetables, and legumes. It can be digested by the body when consumed, and helps to lower blood sugar and cholesterol levels.

Insoluble fiber, which is found in whole wheat, whole grains, celery, corn, corn bran, green beans, green leafy vegetables, potato skins, and brown rice, cannot be digested by the body. Because of this, when you consume it, insoluble fiber does not register as calories—and in fact, the foods that contain them are automatically 15 percent lower in calories than they appear to be. Insoluble fiber also acts as a fat vacuum because when insoluble fiber exists in the body, some of the fat in your digestive system clings to the rough surface of the fiber and exits right along with it.

In addition, insoluble fiber gives the stool needed volume and helps to prevent constipation and possibly eventual colon and rectal cancer.

How Do You Know You're Not Consuming Too Many Calories?

If you keep to the lower or even the middle of the food allowances, I promise you that you will not be consuming too many calories. Depending upon your present weight, height, and metabolism, the higher end may be too high for you. To be on the safe side, try to stick to the middle or lower end of the food allowances until you reach your fitness goal.

Caffeine

When it comes to caffeine, it's up to you. It all depends upon your medical condition and your ability to tolerate caffeine. Caffeine's reputation varies from year to year. Some studies claim that in moderation, it increases energy and is good for your heart. Other studies claim that it's bad for your heart and causes a host of problems from fibrocystic breast disease to raised cholesterol levels. You should discuss your particular situation with your doctor.

I used to be able to drink two to three cups of regular coffee a day. Lately, I find that drinking that amount of coffee makes me jumpy, so I've switched to the "light" coffee with half the amount of caffeine. I can still have my two to three cups, and I no longer feel "hyper." You'll have to pay attention to your body to see if caffeine is friendly to your body, and in what amounts.

Alcohol

Although many studies indicate that up to two glasses of wine a day can in fact be beneficial to your health, I would not drink every day. Why? If nothing else, alcohol consumption, even light alcohol, such as wine or light beer, temporarily slows down your metabolism, and you burn less fat.

If you're going to indulge, save it for the weekend and have one to two drinks one day, or the most, two drinks two days. Such drinking will not retard your fat loss, even if you are on the strictest regimen. But remember to indulge only in the low-calorie nonmixed drinks such as white or red wine, light beer, or liquor with plain soda, water, or, at worst, fruit juice. You may count each drink as a fruit, but remember, you're not getting the nutrition of a fruit.

Salt or Sodium

The human body needs a certain amount of sodium for good health, but not nearly as much as most people consume. The minimum daily requirement for sodium is between 1,500 and 2,400 milligrams, but most people consume as much as double that amount. How so? One serving of full-sodium soup has about 1,000 grams per serving. All full-sodium canned vegetables also have that amount, and most frozen dinners are just as bad. Other high-sodium foods are Chinese food, smoked foods, and all pickled foods—including, of course, my favorite: pickles!

Sodium will not make you fat. It will just make you feel fat and indeed look fatter in the mirror. Why? Sodium holds up to fifty times its weight in water. When you indulge in high-sodium foods you will temporarily retain water—which will make your scale weight go up one to even ten pounds.

But what about health? My motto is, if possible, "Everything in moderation." However, if you don't have a health problem such as high blood pressure, like me, with your doctor's permission you may occasionally want to indulge in high-sodium low-fat foods such as pickles, full-sodium soups, and so on. The way I see it, if it's going to prevent me from eating full-fat cream cheese, I'd rather eat pickles! In fact, I've devised a great sandwich that makes me feel as if I've had a feast. I take a bagel, cut it in half, and load it with sliced pickle, tomato, and onion. Then I go to town. Even now, as I write this, my mouth is watering for such a treat. And you know what? It only has about one gram of fat! Sure, I pay the price of being bloated for a day or two, but once I go back to moderate sodium intake, in a few days the bloat goes down.

The point is you can't get fat by eating high-sodium foods—you can only look fat, but that will go away in a few days from the time you lower your sodium intake!

Calcium

Calcium is the most important mineral when it comes to the maintenance of bones. Most doctors agree that 1,500 milligrams of calcium daily is a healthy minimum amount for women of every age, and especially for women over thirty. The following foods are perfect for natural calcium consumption.

Food Item	Serving	Calcium Content
Yogurt, plain, nonfat	1 cup	452
Yogurt, plain, low fat	1 cup	415
Milk, skim	1 cup	302
Milk, 1 percent	1 cup	300
Mozzarella cheese, part skim	1 oz.	207
Ricotta cheese, part skim	4 oz.	335
Cottage cheese, 1 percent	4 oz.	69
Broccoli	1 cup	100
Collard greens	1 cup	300
Turnip greens	1 cup	200
Kale	1 cup	206
Swiss chard	1 cup	128
Orange juice, calcium fortified	1 cup	300
Soybeans	1 cup	131
Tofu, soft	4 oz.	108
Sardines with bones	3 oz.	372
Lima or kidney beans	1/2 cup	48
Ocean perch	4 oz.	156

Note: Cottage cheese is not considered as good a calcium source as other dairy products.

Get a copy of my book *Bone Building Body Shaping Workout* (see Bibliography) for a list of many other sources of calcium. If you are not sure that you're getting enough calcium in your diet, see your doctor about taking a supplement. But remember, it's always better to get your calcium from food. I never took a calcium supplement in my life, and my bone thickness was measured at 219.3—almost double the thickness of "normal" women my age, and thicker than an average twenty-five-year-old's. Why are my bones so thick? I do my own workouts, and I get my calcium from natural sources.

Drinking Water Helps You Not to Retain Water!

In Chapter 2 we discussed water in the context of its importance in allowing the kidneys the freedom to do their fat-processing work. Now we will see how drinking lots of water actually helps you to flush out excess water from your system.

When your body gets less water than it needs, it goes into a survival mode and begins to retain any bit of water it does get, even the water from foods. This water is stored in the extracellular spaces (outside of the cells) and can actually be seen in your hands, feet, and legs (they will appear swollen). Taking "water pills" (diuretics) is absolutely not the answer because the body goes on red alert and feels that it is being robbed of its life-sustaining water. Then the moment you stop taking the water pills, your body retains every bit of water it can—and you have to wait about a week for it to level off. (It levels off only if you don't eat high-sodium foods.)

So what's the answer? Drink lots of water. But how does water help to flush water out of your system? As the water passes through the kidneys, it takes any excess sodium—and water—with it!

If you drink lots of water, you will also look and feel better. Your skin won't look saggy; it will look firm and healthy. But more than that, water helps to flush out waste from your system and relieve constipation!

How much water should you drink? Six eight-ounce glasses a day would be just fine, even eight if you can swing it. I know it isn't easy—and you'll probably be finding yourself going to the bathroom a lot—but it's well worth it.

Eat Often!

You'll lose more weight if you eat five small meals a day, even if those meals add up to more calories than one big meal! Why? When you break up your eating, you give your body the energy it needs to function, and it does not go into the "survival" stage and slow down your metabolism—which in turn causes you, all things being equal, to burn less calories.

The only way to lose weight and keep it off is to prevent the body from feeling deprived. You must gently coax your body into letting go of its excess fat by giving it food all day long. The trick is, instead of giving it fatty foods, you give it nutritious low-fat foods in a well-balanced diet (as listed above). Your body will cooperate with you fully because it was created to eat a well-balanced diet.

If, on the other hand, you try to go against nature and punish your body for being fat, telling it "You will not eat all day, you fat pig," and then at the end of the day give it some food, your body will rebel and sabotage you and force you to eat much more than you had planned. Clearly, then, for two reasons, slowed metabolism and sabotage, you must eat often. Five or more times a day is ideal, but three is the bare, bare minimum.

Once You Reach Your Goal, Eat Anything You Want One Day a Week!

There's a pot of gold at the end of the rainbow! Once you reach your goal, you can eat anything you want, all day long, once a week. "But how could this work?" you might ask. By consuming a well-balanced low-fat diet all week long, you make room for the additional fat intake on the free day. In other words, it evens out! But how can you be sure that you won't gain weight if you do that? Think of it logically. For six days you are eating a low-fat diet. One day you eat high fat. Yes. It's one step forward and one step back, which leads you right to where you are now: maintenance of what you have, in other words.

The fact is, if you continued to follow the low-fat, balanced eating plan in this chapter for the rest of your life, never taking a free eating day even when you reached your ideal body weight, you would eventually lose too much weight and you would begin to appear too thin.

When I first tried this out, I planned my eating day all week. Every time I thought of a goody that I was missing, I would write it down, and then when I was in the supermarket, I would purchase the item: Cheez-Its, Tootsie Rolls, full-fat ice cream, full-fat cream cheese, lox, a juicy red steak, and so on. Then when my free eating day came, I got up early in the morning and started my day with a fatty lox and cream cheese bagel. I continued to eat all day, and was in fact annoyed that at times I was too stuffed to eat—and even felt slightly nauseous. By the end of the day, or should I say night, I was upset that I couldn't fit in those last few full-fat gingerbread cookies!

The next day I'd feel horrible. I had a headache, a stomachache, and even a backache. I ate well all week, and when the next week came, I just ate what I pleased instead of going out of my way to "get it all in."

Why did I tell you this? I wanted you to know that it is okay to go through your crazy stage. Don't worry. Your own body will help to level you off. And the beauty of it is that, with this plan, you soon lose your sense of depression. You realize that there's no emergency. If you don't get to eat that goody you've been craving this week, you can always have it next week.

A free eating day! What a wonderful gift. If I didn't have it, I don't think I would be motivated to keep to a low-fat eating plan, knowing that for the rest of my life I would have no reward coming to me.

But what happens if you slip and start taking two or more free eating days—and, say, you start gaining weight? Fine. Just go back on the full low-fat eating plan until you are again at your goal. Then take your free eating day once a week again. In order to prevent weight gain, a good rule of thumb is, any free eating day over one a week will cost you an extra week of not taking a free eating day. In other words, if you pig out on the holidays for five days in a row, then don't take a free eating day for five weeks. It's that simple—and it works. (For other options for free eating, like having one small goody a day, see my diet book *Eat to Trim* in Bibliography.)

In Summary: The Basic Food Rules to Follow

1. Eat your minimum for the day: 2–3 servings of protein; 6–10 servings of limited complex carbohydrates; 3–12 or more servings of vegetables; 2–4 fruits; 1–2 servings of dairy. (Except for the vegetable category, which works in reverse, the closer you keep to the lower allotment, the faster you will lose your excess fat.)

2. Eat often—five times a day or more. Never go more than four hours without eating!

3. Drink lots of water. Drink six to eight glasses of water a day. You can have a glass first thing in the morning, one before each meal, and one during or after exercising.

4. When you reach your fitness goal, eat anything you want once a week.

5. High-fat foods are public enemy number one, but high-sugar foods are potential menaces to fat loss. High-sodium foods will not make you fat—they will make you *look* fat for a short time! Be aware.

Make Your Own Meal Plans

Using the above guide, here is a sample meal plan:

Breakfast	Fat Grams	Calories
1/2 cup hot cereal (1cc #1) with 1 cup 1% milk (d #1)	2 milk, 1 cereal	150 cereal 100 milk
1 orange (f #1) No-calorie drink	0 orange	69

Snack	Fat Grams	Calories
4 oz. nonfat cottage cheese (d #2)	0 cottage cheese	80

Lunch

	Fat Grams	Calories
6 oz. flounder (p #1)	3.2 flounder	120
and 1 cup rice (1cc #2 and 3)	1 rice	200
large tossed lettuce and tomato salad (v #2,3,4)	0 salad	50

Snack

	Fat Grams	Calories
4 low-fat crackers (lcc #4)	1 cracker	48
1/2 grapefruit (f #2)	0 grapefruit	46

Dinner

	Fat Grams	Calories
6 oz. broiled chicken (p #2)	7.5 chicken	192
1 cup broccoli and cauliflower (v #5 and 6)	0 vegetables	50
2/3 cup pasta, with 1/2 cup low-fat tomato sauce (lcc #5 and 6)	1 pasta, 6 tomato sauce	200 50

Snack

	Fat Grams	Calories
2 cups brussels sprouts and carrots (v #7–10)	0 vegetables	130

Note: The code for each nutritional requirement is in parentheses. v = vegetables; lcc = limited complex carbohydrates; f = fruit; p = protein; and d = dairy.

Now let's count it up and see if we have filled the bill for a nutritionally healthy diet, and, at the same time, a low-fat diet.

3–12 or more servings of vegetables

6–10 servings of limited complex carbohydrates

2–4 fruits

2–3 servings of protein

2–3 servings of dairy

You've consumed twenty-three grams of fat—under your maximum—and only 1,485 calories, and look at all the food you ate. You had two servings of protein, opting for the six-ounce servings instead of the four-ounce, but keeping to the two instead of the three servings. You had six limited complex carbohydrates—the lower end of the allowance—and two fruits—again the lower end of the allowance. You had two dairys—the higher end of the allowance—and you had ten servings of vegetables, a good amount more than the bare minimum—exactly what I want you to do. But what if you were still hungry?

You would have two options: (1) eat more vegetables from the unlimited complex carbohydrate group; or (2) go closer to the higher end of your food allowance. It is much better to use option number one if your goal is to lose the most weight in the least amount of time. If you choose to eat toward the higher end of your food allowance, you will still lose weight in time, but it will take a little longer. But so what? I don't want you to feel deprived. Better to keep to the higher end than to blow your diet and start eating fatty foods in rebellion, in which case, in time, you'll only be fatter!

Note: For a much more complete diet with a whole month's worth of meal plans (three meals and two snacks a day—easy recipes, and you never repeat a meal), send for a copy of *Eat to Trim*. See Bibliography.

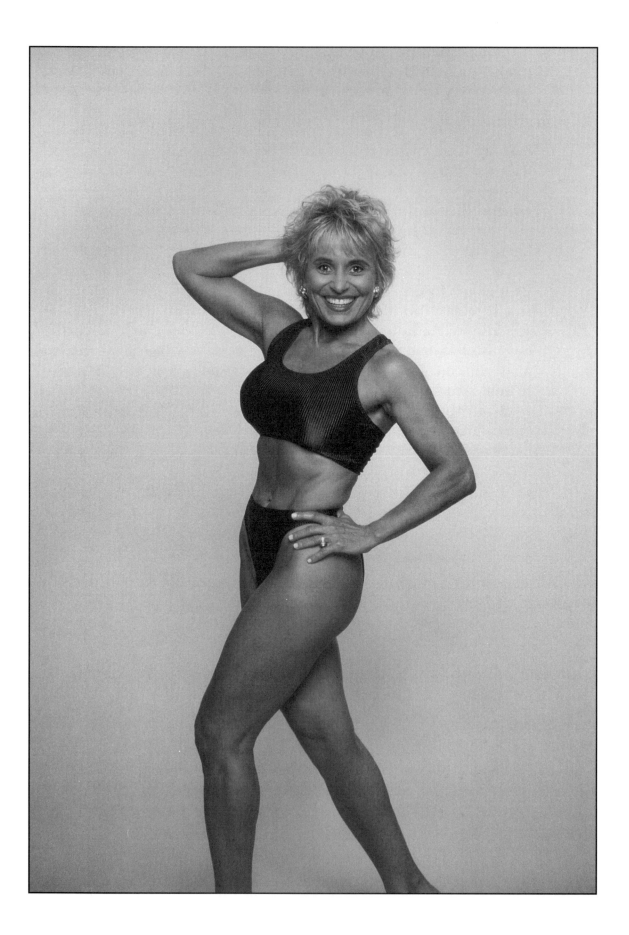

8

EXTRA FAT-BURNING TECHNIQUES

You can't burn enough fat. You probably feel that way, at least if you love to eat as much as I do! In this chapter, I'll share some of my additional fat-burning techniques, methods I've discovered that help to burn extra calories during a given day, so that you can eat more than you would otherwise be able to eat—and still stay lean and sexy. First we'll talk about aerobics in general, and the amount of fat that can be burned doing various activities for a given amount of time. Then we'll discuss specific aerobic activities, detailing the advantages of each and describing the specific muscles utilized. Finally, we'll talk about simple ways to stimulate the metabolism during a typical day so that yet more fat can be burned in a relatively painless way.

Aerobic Activities

First of all, I must point out that in order to burn fat, an exercise does not have to be aerobic. As long as you are alive, you are using calories and burning fat. However, if you were going to depend upon just breathing to burn fat, your fat-burning rate would be very slow—because most people burn only about forty to sixty calories an hour just breathing. So what's the most time-efficient way of burning fat? Although it will not sculpt your body, aerobic exercise will burn the most calories in the shortest amount of time.

But what is aerobic? Literally, the word means "with oxygen." Although all exercise, indeed all life, requires oxygen, exercise is considered aerobic when it causes your pulse to reach a rate of 60 to 85 percent of its capacity, and to maintain that elevated rate for a certain length of time, usually twenty or more minutes. In the following paragraphs you will find a description of various aerobic exercises in order of most fat-burning to least fat-burning.

I can guess what you may be thinking. "Great. I'll just look at the top of the chart and pick the most fat-burning of all the activities." That may or may not be a good idea! It's much better to pick an exercise that you enjoy so you will look forward to working out. If you don't enjoy your exercise, you'll probably feel defeated; you won't want to work out, and you may find that even the thought of the exercise robs you of your will to live, much less work out. I know that feeling—believe me!

In other words, while one fat-burning activity may be more "aerobic" than another (burn more fat in a given period of time) and although you may be perfectly capable of performing that activity, if you hate it, you are setting yourself up for failure. It's just not worth it.

Before we begin our discussion of aerobic workouts, I want to point out that the Bathing Suit Workout is aerobic if you don't take your optional rests—and even if you do, it is partially aerobic. If you only have limited time and have to choose "either/or"—that is to say, the Bathing Suit Workout or one of the aerobic workouts listed in this chapter—by all means, choose the Bathing Suit Workout! However, if you have the time (and I hope you *make* the time) it's a good idea to perform additional fat-burning aerobic activities.

As mentioned in Chapter 4, when performing a fat-burning aerobic activity, the goal is to get your heart rate up to between 60 and 70 percent of its capacity. You could go higher—as high as 80 to 85 percent of capacity. However, most fitness experts agree that the ideal fat-burning range is the lower range of 60 to 70 percent of capacity. In addition, working at this lower heart rate enables most people to work out for longer periods of time if they choose to do so—and in the end, burn more fat.

By way of review, in order to tell whether you are in the fat-burning range, subtract your age from the number 220 and then multiply that by 60 percent. This will be your basement fat-burning range. To calculate the higher ranges, simply multiply the 220 figure by 65 percent, 70 percent, and so on.

I'll use myself as an example. I'm fifty-five years old. If I subtract 55 from 220, I get 165. Now I multiply that number by 60 percent. The answer is 99.0. So when I measure my pulse rate for one minute after doing a given exercise for at least seven minutes and my pulse beats 99 times, I know that I am in my fat-burning range of about 60 percent. If my pulse beats, say, 115 times in a minute, I'm in the 70 percent range (70 percent of 165 is 115.5).

All well and good. But how do you find *your* pulse, and then how do you calculate *your* percentage? Luckily, you don't have to count your pulse for an entire minute. You can do it for fifteen seconds and multiply the number by four instead. Place your fingers on your wrist and feel around until you can feel a pulse. Then set a stopwatch or look at the second hand of your watch for fifteen seconds while you count the beats. When you get a final figure, multiply it by four. For example, if my fifteen-second rate were 26 and I multiplied it by 4, I would have a total of 104. I would know that I was working at 60 percent of my capacity. If it were higher, say 30, the total would be 120—and I would know that I was in the 70 percent range.

If you get a headache just thinking about all this calculating and monitoring, you can do what I do. Instead of counting, just notice whether you are breaking into a mild sweat after about seven minutes. If you are, you are in the fat-burning range. If you're not, work a little harder. Move faster, flex your muscles—whatever it takes to give it that extra bit of effort.

Aerobic Fat-Burning Chart

Aerobic Activity	Calories Burned per 20 Minutes
Running an eight-minute mile (outdoors or on a treadmill)	230
Running a nine-minute mile (outdoors or on a treadmill)	220
Cross-country skiing	220
Swimming	210
Box aerobics (Boxercise)	200
Step aerobics	200
Stair-stepping	200
Rope jumping	200
Low-impact aerobics (aerobic dance)	200
NordicTrack machine	165
Trampoline jumping	165
Racewalking	160
Hiking (hills)	160
Rowing machine	150
Jogging at a slow pace (outdoors or on a treadmill)	145
Bicycle riding (stationary or moving at moderate pace)	140
Pool aerobics and water walking	140
Dancing at quick pace	120
Walking at a quick pace (outdoors or on a treadmill)	110

The above chart is a generalization for people of medium height and weight. If you are a big person, you will burn more calories than above. If you are a small person, you may burn a little less than the chart above, but you can compensate for that by moving faster and flexing your muscles as you work.

How Many Minutes Should You Work Out?

The ideal time is twenty to forty-five minutes. Can you go shorter or longer? Of course. Most fitness experts agree that even eight to ten minutes of aerobics is a lot better than nothing. But what about going longer—say, an hour?

I don't think it's a good idea as a general rule. If you try to do aerobics for sixty minutes at a session, you may overtrain your body and become fatigued. In addition, you will probably find yourself dreading the next aerobic workout. Remember, you're in this for the long term. It's much better to do short, enjoyable aerobic activities over a sustained period of time than to do one or two killer workouts that destroy your morale.

When I do aerobics, I work out from twenty to forty-five minutes, depending upon how strenuous the exercise. When I'm leisurely riding the exercise bike, I'll do up to forty-five minutes. But when I'm running, I run for about twenty minutes. If I walk, on the other hand, I can go for a full hour.

What? Didn't I just contradict myself? No. You see, since walking at a brisk pace is the least strenuous aerobic activity (in fact it is considered by some to be near-aerobic, not strictly aerobic) you can do it longer than other aerobic activities without becoming exhausted.

How Many Days a Week Should You Do Aerobics?

If possible, in addition to your Bathing Suit Workout and/or other weight-training workout, you should do aerobics four to five days a week. If you want to do less, three days is fine. If you want to do more, take a day off after six to ten days—preferably after six days.

You can do your aerobics on the same days you do your Bathing Suit Workout and/or other weight-training workout (you'll have to do that if you are doing aerobics more than three days a week), or you can do your aerobics on the days you don't do your Bathing Suit Workout and/or other weight-training workout.

When Should You Do Aerobics—Before or after Your Bathing Suit Workout or Other Weight-Training Workout?

In other books, I've always said, "Do your aerobic activity when it suits you best. It doesn't really matter." But after careful experimentation, I must tell you that if your schedule allows, it's always better to do your aerobics first, and your weight-training workout immediately after. The aerobic activity seems to provide an energy burst that lasts for about forty minutes, so why not take advantage of that energy and use it to do your Bathing Suit Workout and/or other weight-training-type workout?

But wait a minute. I'm still wary about encouraging you to do your aerobics first. Why? It is the Bathing Suit Workout that is most important. I'm afraid that you may say to yourself, "Well, I did my aerobics—and I just don't have time to invest in my Bathing Suit Workout (and/or other weight-training-type workout)." That would be the biggest mistake you could make. So if it comes down to either/or and you are pressed for time, do your Bathing Suit Workout first.

The best idea is to get used to your Bathing Suit Workout first. Make it an essential part of your life, like brushing your teeth or taking a shower. After you've established the workout habit, then, if you choose to do your aerobics first, I'm not worried that you'll be tempted to cut out the most important workout.

How Can You Break In to Aerobics if You've Never Done Aerobics Before?

The following schedule applies to all aerobic activities except brisk walking, which can be done ten to twenty minutes a day for the first week, and then adding ten to twenty minutes a week until you reach your goal. For all other aerobic activities, the following chart applies.

Week 1: Three to five minutes

Week 2: Five to seven minutes

Week 3: Seven to ten minutes

Week 4: Ten to fifteen minutes

Week 5: Fifteen to twenty minutes

Week 6: Twenty to twenty-five minutes

Week 7: Twenty-five to thirty minutes

Week 8: Thirty to thirty-five minutes

Week 9: Thirty-five to forty minutes

Week 10: Forty to forty-five minutes

Can you build up to your maximum amount more quickly than the above chart? Yes. With your doctor's permission, you can probably double your time, but be sure to check with him or her.

In any case, begin at the lower end of each week's range and work your way upward, so at the end of the week you are doing the higher number. For example, if you're jumping rope, on the first day of Week 1 you will jump rope for three minutes. The second time you jump rope that week, you will go for four minutes. The last few times you jump rope, you will go for five minutes.

Breaking In to a New Aerobic Activity if You're Already in Aerobic Shape with Another Aerobic Activity

What if you are already in aerobic shape for, say, using the stair machine, but now you want to try rope jumping? You are used to using the stair machine for twenty minutes with no problem. So you think, "I'll just jump rope today for twenty minutes." But after three minutes you are shocked to see that you are out of breath. "What's wrong with me?" you wonder. Perhaps rope jumping is much harder than stair-stepping.

Wrong. Had you been a rope-jumper and tried to switch to stair-stepping, you would probably have felt the same way. One aerobic activity is different from another, because different muscles are emphasized. For example, when you stair-step, you use your lower body muscles in a pumping motion, whereas when you jump rope, you use lower body muscles in a springing motion. In addition, in rope-jumping your upper body comes into play.

No matter which aerobic activity you are switching to, it takes a little while to make the transition. How much time? It all depends upon you. Happily, it will not take nearly as long as the regular break-in-gently program if you are already in aerobic shape. Here is a guideline. As above, you may break in twice as fast if you are able to do so and, of course, with your doctor's permission.

Week 1: Five to ten minutes

Week 2: Ten to fifteen minutes

Week 3: Fifteen to twenty-five minutes

Week 4: Twenty-five to forty-five minutes

Specific Aerobic Activities

Which aerobic exercise you choose will depend upon your particular interest and ability. For example, I hate the water, so I would never choose swimming. I love running but my joints hurt, so I can only do that twice a week at the most. So what I like is not always what I can do. My second choice for aerobics is either riding the stationary bike or doing the stair-stepper or, better yet, walking at a brisk pace.

The ideal thing is to switch around and do various aerobic activities in a given week. For example, if I'm going to do aerobics five times a week, I run twice, ride the bike twice, and do the stair-stepper once. I may do that for a few weeks and then replace the running with jumping rope. A few weeks later I may replace the bike with trampoline jumping. On weeks when I have a swing dance lesson, I use the sixty-minute lesson as one aerobic session.

What if you want to do the same aerobic activity every day? Fine with me. You'll still burn fat and get your heart and lungs in shape. Bear in mind, however, that after a while your body might appreciate some variety. It will give other muscles a chance to be involved and will round out your overall endurance.

No matter which aerobic activity you choose, remember that the key is to enjoy yourself and at the same time burn excess fat and get your heart and lungs into top shape. If you find yourself dreading your aerobic activity, give yourself a break and take the time to explore others. If you're a creature of habit, in the beginning you may fight the idea, thinking "I may not get as much out of it" or "This will be too hard." But you'll be surprised to see that after a week or two you'll feel as if you've been doing the activity forever.

RUNNING OUTDOORS OR ON A TREADMILL

For me, running outdoors is one of the most enjoyable ways of exercising. You breathe fresh air and at the same time watch the scenes of nature as you go. After the first few minutes, you find yourself thinking, solving problems, or just letting your mind run free. In addition, running seems to give the highest of natural highs. I tell you, it is almost impossible to remain sad or depressed after having a great run.

Unfortunately, running outdoors can put a strain on your joints and eventually cause problems. For example, I started running about fifteen years ago. In the beginning I overdid it, trying to use running as a way to get in shape (before I knew what I know now). I ended up with shin splints and knee problems. Later I purchased the proper running shoes and began running mainly on grass or dirt—and cut my running time to thirty minutes instead of an hour. But still, in time, the running became a problem. At night my knee and hip joints would ache; I would feel a grinding sensation. So I experimented by cutting out running for three months. Sure enough, the pain went away. "I'll see what happens if I run only twice a week," I said. And I did and it worked fine.

But I didn't leave it at that. I decided to see what would happen if I ran three or four days a week again. Sure enough, in two months the pain was back. Again I stopped for three months. After that I made it a rule: Never, no matter what, run more than two days a week—and I'm fine. No problem.

What about running on a treadmill? Is it the same as running outdoors? Yes and no. If you raise your feet off the ground and "spring" the way you must do on the real ground, it is the same. However, if you move as quickly as you would if you were running but take advantage of the sliding surface of the treadmill and don't spring off the ground, you save your joints from the shock of the bounce.

Running on a treadmill has another advantage. You can adjust the speed and incline of the "floor," making the run harder or easier depending upon your needs. In addition, most treadmills have monitors that will tell you, depending upon your weight, sex, age, and height, exactly how many calories you are burning for a given time period.

Why don't I switch to the treadmill? I hate it! To me it's boring, even if you put flying country scenes on a screen in front of me. Also, I can't help but feeling like the proverbial rat on a wheel, scurrying madly and going nowhere. But don't let my feelingsg stop you. I have many friends who love the treadmill and in fact use it as their main aerobic activity, burning much fat and getting their hearts and lungs in top shape.

CROSS-COUNTRY SKIING

If you don't mind cold weather and love the snow, cross-country skiing can be a wonderful aerobic activity. Unlike downhill skiing where once you glide down the hill you must stop and wait to ascend the hill on a lift, in cross-country or Nordic skiing, you are continually on the move. What's more, depending upon where you live, cross-country skiing can be done right outside your door. In fact, I've seen cross-country skiers in the streets of Manhattan—yes, Manhattan—during winters when there have been continual heavy snowstorms.

With this activity, you use not only your lower-body muscles—calves, thighs, hips, buttocks, and abdominals—but your upper-body muscles as well—back, chest, shoulders, and arms.

SWIMMING

The most body-gentle aerobic activity is swimming. When you swim, you put almost no pressure at all on your bones or joints. In fact, when an athlete sustains an injury and wishes to remain in shape, the first thing most doctors will recommend is swimming. In fact, years ago, when I used to be a judo player, I tore the cartilage in my knee. After about six weeks of complete layoff, my knee was still not in condition to even walk more than the minimum amount, much less run. My doctor recommended swimming.

As much as I hate the water, I dragged myself to the pool every day. At the time I was teaching in a high school where there was a pool. I would arrive every day at 6 A.M. and swim back and forth from one end of the shallow side to the other. (I have a fear of deep water and finally realized that swimming alone was not the way to overcome it.)

I thought that in time I would come to love the water. But in spite of the fact that I was forced to swim for four months, I'll never forget the first long walk I took without pain! I felt as if my life were given back to me. I never went near the water again! I'm just not a water person.

Notwithstanding my personal preferences, swimming is excellent exercise. It involves all the muscles in the body, but there is a greater emphasis on upper-body muscles—back, chest, shoulders, and arms are involved—and in fact even the neck comes into play. Of course you also use your thighs and hips/buttocks area. The calves are hardly involved at all.

BOX AEROBICS (BOXERCISE)

Box aerobics or boxercise can be great fun, and at the same time it provides an outlet for stress, aggression, and anger. In addition, this exercise can increase ability in self-defense and, with it, self-confidence and even self-esteem. The workout consists of a jumping movement with punches and jabs, and sometimes includes the punching of a "heavybag," and a little rope jumping. Women who engage in this exercise tell me that every time they boxercise they leave the exercise room feeling transformed.

Boxercise works all of the upper-body muscles—back, chest, shoulders, arms—as well as the lower-body muscles—calves, thighs, hips/buttocks, and abdominals. You gain muscle strength, coordination, and skill in self-defense, all at the same time. I love this exercise.

STEP AEROBICS

If you are fairly coordinated and enjoy working out with people, step aerobics can be fun. You get to key into the energy of the group, especially the step-aerobics leader, who usually has enough energy to fuel a battleship!

The one drawback I find with step aerobics is that you must "learn" something. In other words, unlike simply getting on a treadmill or paddling away in the water (assuming you know how to swim), you must learn the sometimes complicated steps the instructor is doing. Most step-aerobics teachers provide classes for beginners so that newcomers don't become discouraged from the start. In time, most people surprise themselves and are able to keep up with even the most advanced step-aerobics sessions. I don't like step aerobics. To me, no matter how many fancy steps they throw in, it's tedious. But to each her own. I know women who live for this exercise.

Step aerobics provides most of its work for the lower body, specifically the calves, thighs, and hips/buttock area, as well as the abdominals. Can you reshape these body parts with step aerobics? Not in a million years. What you will do is strengthen them by the repeated motion. In order to do ultimate reshaping, you must work in sets and repetitions and, ideally, with graduated weights.

STAIR-STEPPING

There are a variety of stair-stepping machines ranging from the kind featuring elaborate devices that enable you to increase the incline and the tension of the "climb" to those with no high-tech controls at all.

If you choose to do stair-stepping, you don't need the fancy devices. But make sure you do break into a sweat after about seven minutes. I've seen people on these machines working out for forty-five minutes and not break into a sweat. The watch TV or read a book and barely move their legs, all the time thinking, "I'm really working out."

To avoid this pitfall, when stair stepping, pump hard and make sure you don't shorten the "stepping" movement to just two or three inches. Go the full range (six to ten inches), and flex your thighs and/or hips/buttocks muscles as you go. If you squeeze your working buttock on each descent, you will put more emphasis on that area. On the other hand, if you flex your working thigh muscle with each down movement, you'll put more emphasis there. And if you flex both your thighs and your hips/buttock muscles as you go, you'll get the most aerobic workout for your exercise time. It isn't easy—you'll find yourself wanting to just forget about flexing and enjoy yourself. You can do that as long as you are sweating. But if you're not, you'll have to put in the extra effort.

Stair-stepping works mainly your lower body: calves, thighs, hips/buttocks, and abdominals. The upper-body muscles are not really involved, except for a little lower-back work.

ROPE JUMPING

Rope jumping can be lots of fun. You can do it at home while watching TV, or out in your backyard while gazing at the birds, flowers, trees, sun, and sky. You can also use rope jumping as an aerobic activity in your hotel room while on vacation or on a business trip. I do it whenever I'm on the road. In fact, rope jumping saves me the time and effort of waiting for a free exercise bike if there is a workout room, or of walking or running around a strange neighborhood early in the morning—something I'm not always in the mood to do. Knowing that I can do my aerobic workout in the privacy of my own room helps me to look forward to getting up in the morning instead of dreading the ring of that telephone wake-up call.

Rope jumping involves both lower- and upper-body muscles. You use your calves, thighs, hips, and buttocks, as well as your abdominal muscles, as you jump. At the same time, you use your back, chest, shoulders, and arms as you swing the rope around with every step. If you like rope jumping, after a while you can begin to vary your steps, doing fancy quick combinations the way fighters do when they train. In fact, at some health spas they have rope-jumping classes where you can really learn to get fancy. But you don't have to go to that extreme. I find that just the basic jump gives me quite a workout.

LOW-IMPACT AEROBICS (AEROBIC DANCE)

If you love music and have rhythm, aerobic dance can be the most painless aerobic activity in the world. When you do it to great music with a reasonable instructor who keeps it simple enough for you to follow, you lose track of time. Before you know it, twenty or more minutes have flown by and the session is over. You can't believe your workout is finished.

If you do aerobic dance, you'll find that if you choose a class where the music suits your temperament, you'll be much more motivated to move. For example, if I go to a class where they're playing disco-type music, which offends my sensibilities, I find myself slugging away, watching the clock and wishing it were over with. On the other hand, if I choose a class that features jazz-type music, or music from the fifties, I work out with so much enthusiasm and energy that I'm actually surprised and disappointed when the class ends. What's more, I'm in such a great mood when it's over that I can't help but start conversations with the next five people I meet.

Aerobic dance involves the entire body. You're using your lower body to propel you—calves, thighs, hips/buttocks, and abdominals—and at the same time you're using your upper body—back, chest, shoulders, and arms—in rhythm to the music. It's a great total-body workout.

Note: Be sure to choose "low-impact" aerobic dance as opposed to "high-impact," where you leap off the ground and land hard. This can cause eventual damage to your bones and joints.

NORDICTRACK MACHINE AND OTHER SIMILAR MACHINES

The NordicTrack machine can provide an excellent total-body workout. While it of course can't reshape any body part, it can help you to increase your overall body strength and endurance. The great thing about this machine is that it can be purchased at a reasonable price and kept in the corner of a room at home. You can do it while watching TV listening to music, or just thinking. If you don't want to purchase such a machine, you can find one in most fitness centers.

This machine mimics the motion of cross-country skiing, which is handy if you live in a climate with no snow. It allows you to use both lower- and upper-body muscles in a challenging way. Your calves, thighs, hips/buttocks, and abdominals are working as you perform the skilike motion, while at the same time your back, chest, shoulders, and arms are being challenged as you simulate the movement you would make with ski poles.

TRAMPOLINE JUMPING

Trampoline jumping can be lots of fun if you do it to music. It's a real gift for those who would like to jump rope but can't do so because they live in an apartment building and would disturb neighbors by jumping directly on the floor. What's more, trampolines come in small sizes now and can be stored under a bed or behind a piece of furniture.

When you jump on a trampoline, make up your own routines. March for a while, then just plain jump high with both feet, then do a skipping motion, and so on. Try to use your arms. You can move them up and down the way you would if you were walking at a fast pace, punch into the air as if you were boxing an imaginary opponent, or clap them over your head as if you were doing jumping jacks.

Depending upon how you work, the trampoline can exercise your entire body. No matter what you do, you will be exercising your calves, thighs, hips/buttocks, and abdominals. If you employ the above upper-body techniques, you'll also be using your back, chest, shoulders, and arms.

RACEWALKING

If you love to run but can't do it for health reasons, racewalking is your second-best bet—and it's quite a challenge. In order for your activity to be considered true racewalking, you must move very fast—almost as fast as a runner—but without springing off the ground the way runners do. Experienced racewalkers can in fact outpace some runners.

If racewalking has any disadvantage, I would say it's the way people look when they do it. I've never seen a racewalker who in my eyes, didn't look, well, foolish! They seem to be jerking forward in an unnatural, almost robotic, way. Why do they look this way? In order to racewalk properly, you must maintain high muscle tension and an as-rapid-as-possible pace. In addition, at the same time you must move your arms back and forth with each step in a rigid marchlike motion.

If I liked to racewalk, I wouldn't let the way I looked stop me. Who cares what people think? If they're not paying your rent, I say forget about people and enjoy yourself.

If performed properly, this exercise utilizes all the muscles in the body: calves, thighs, hips/buttocks, abdominals, back, chest, shoulders, and arms.

HIKING (HILLS)

Hiking is one of my favorite activities because it is done out of doors and you can lose yourself in nature. In fact, when I hike, I don't know I'm working out at all, and I can do it for hours at a time. I especially love hiking in Arizona, where I can take in the view of the cacti and the canyons. It fills my soul with joy and I remember it for months afterwards. Also, hiking is an activity that you can do either by yourself or with others. I like to hike with a group of people. Often I find that we don't speak for long periods of time, each of us absorbed in experiencing nature. Yet we seem to be communicating anyway, because when we do speak, we seem to start in the middle of a conversation, yet no one is confused. Apparently we were all tuned in to nature and on the same wavelength.

If you're going to hike, be sure that you do it where the ground is not always completely flat because you won't get as much out of it. Find a place where there are hilly spots as well as flat terrain. If you can't find hilly spots, then walk faster and try to flex your muscles as you go.

Hiking utilizes both lower- and upper-body muscles if you do it right. You use your calves, thighs, hips/buttocks, and abdominals as you propel yourself along, and you use your back, chest, shoulders, and arms if you make a conscious effort to do so.

ROWING MACHINE

The rowing machine does exactly what its name states: It simulates the rowing motion. In fact, if you've ever rowed a boat, you'll recognize the feeling as soon as you begin the workout. It isn't easy at first, but once you get used to it you'll surprise yourself with how quickly you build endurance. I remember the first time I tried it. I only lasted seven minutes. But the next time I doubled my workout. By the end of the week, after a fourth try, I was rowing for thirty minutes! Of course, I was already in aerobic shape from other exercises.

Naturally, the rowing machine stresses mainly upper-body muscles: back, chest, shoulders, and arms. You can build a nice amount of upper-body strength doing this exercise. I must remind you, however, that you cannot hope to reshape an upper-body part with this aerobic exercise. You must work out with weights the right way in order to do that! The machine is set up in such a way that your hips, buttocks, and legs are doing a small amount of work, but not enough to build any lower-body strength. The calves are completely left out of the workout.

JOGGING AT A SLOW PACE

Years ago, when running first became popular, whether people ran or jogged they called it "jogging." But over time, the term *jogging* came to mean running at a slow or leisurely pace.

Jogging can be a very relaxing, enjoyable exercise. In fact, it is so relaxing that the people who do it often appear to be half asleep! Every time I see a jogger padding by I have to bite my tongue because I feel like quipping, "Now don't strain yourself." In fact, if you want to know whether you're jogging or running, think of that image. If someone were to see you, would they be tempted to say that to you?

Jogging is the halfway point between walking and running, yet notice that you don't burn as many calories doing it as you would race-walking. Why? When you racewalk, even though your feet don't spring off the ground, you really push it. You're straining every muscle in your body to propel yourself along as quickly as possible without catapulting yourself off the ground. In addition, you're using a marching movement, swinging your bent arms back and forth and flexing your muscles all the time. When you jog, on the other hand, speed is not the issue. Even though you do spring off the ground with each step, you spring in a very leisurely manner. In addition, when you jog, instead of making your arms work as hard as possible, you simply use them naturally.

Jogging employs mainly the lower-body muscles: calves, thighs, hips/buttocks, and abdominals. You do exercise your upper body—back, chest, shoulders and arms—but very lightly. If you have trouble with your bones and joints, just as in running, you will have to keep jogging to a limit, although jogging will provide slightly less stress on bones and joints than running because you are going slowly and not landing as hard. I am too impatient to jog. I'd rather run or walk at a quick pace.

BICYCLE RIDING (STATIONARY OR MOVING AT A MODERATE PACE)

I find riding the stationary bike while watching TV and keeping up with the current talk shows to be a painless way of burning off some excess fat! I keep the tension low and pedal fast. (High tension may wear down hard-earned muscle.) I do it for about double the time I would do a more strenuous aerobic activity. To me it's worth the extra bike-riding time to burn off the same amount of calories because it's so relaxing. (I'll ride for forty minutes whereas if I ran, I would run for only twenty minutes.)

There are many fancy stationary bicycles available. They have monitoring devices that will tell you exactly how many calories you burned in a given time period, what your heart condition is for your age, and whether or not you defeated the computer "competitor." Such devices can be fun and can help the time to go by more quickly. From time to time I like to try them.

Many stationary bicycles have upper-body devices that allow you to move your arms along with your legs, giving you an upper-body workout along with your lower body. If you are already working your upper body with weights, like me, you may find that this addition is superfluous.

Riding the bicycle outdoors provides basically the same exercise as does the stationary bike; however, outdoor riding cannot be as consistent as the stationary bike. When you are outdoors you may have to stop for pedestrians, dogs, traffic lights, obstacles in the road, and so on. On the other hand, outdoor riding can be more pleasurable. You get to breathe in the fresh air and fill your eyes with the wonders of nature. In addition, it can be more challenging, especially if your route includes hills.

Unless you are using the upper-body attachment on a stationary bike, bicycle riding exercises mainly the lower-body muscles, thighs and hips/buttocks, with a little exercise of the calves and abdominals. If you use the upper-body device on a stationary bicycle, you are also working your back, chest, shoulders, and arms.

POOL AEROBICS AND WATER WALKING

Pool aerobics and water walking are done in a group and can be lots of fun if you like the water. Some of the exercises are done in standing or lying positions (on the stomach or back). Others are done walking in the water. Pressure of the water against the working muscle provides the resistance for the workout. This type of exercise is very gentle on your joints, and is ideal for people who have arthritis or injuries and want to work out.

If you don't mind feeling a bit waterlogged and if you like working out in a group, this exercise can be a welcome change of pace. It provides a total-body workout, depending, of course, on the emphasis of the group leader. Back, chest, shoulders, arms, calves, thighs, hips/buttocks, and abdominals should all come into play.

DANCING AT A QUICK PACE

In order to count dancing as an aerobic activity, you'll have to keep it moving. In other words, if you go out socially to dance, you can't sit down—even for one number—until, say, twenty minutes are up. Since I take ballroom dance lessons that are one hour long and we don't stop moving for a minute, I can count my dancing as aerobic. However, I can do so only because the dances I do are quick paced. I do the fox-trot, tango, the peabody, the quick-step, swing, the samba, the mambo, the cha-cha, and the merengue—all fast-paced dances. But even the waltz, when done with fancy steps and energy, can be considered a quick-paced dance.

Most people don't do ballroom dancing, but rather "freestyle" or country and western dances. Freestyle dancing can be perfect for an aerobic workout because you are in complete control of your pace. Your partner is not connected to you. He or she is dancing nearby doing his or her own thing. You can move as quickly and as vigorously as you choose. You can leap up or, if you dare, even go down to the floor—or do anything you please—and get the amount of calorie burning you choose.

Country and western dance is also perfect for quick-paced dancing that burns calories. If you do the two-step with energy or engage in any of the line dances, you are sure to burn a decent amount of fat.

Dancing provides a total-body workout. The lower-body muscles are employed with each step—calves, thighs, hips/buttocks, and abdominals—and the upper-body muscles—back, chest, shoulders, and arms—are moving to the rhythm of the music. And dancing is fun. You don't even think of it as a workout.

WALKING AT A QUICK PACE

Walking is by far the most convenient of all aerobic workouts. You do it anyway, so all you have to do is do it longer and more briskly, and you've got yourself a workout. In addition, you can do it anywhere, and in any clothing. And perhaps the best part is that, when you do it, nobody has to know you're exercising because you look as if you're just walking like anybody else, only you're moving at a brisk pace as if you have business to attend to.

I love to walk. That's when I do some of my best thinking. Whenever possible, I go early in the morning, at the crack of dawn. I smell the freshly cut grass and the fragrance of the flowers and trees and look at the cloud formations in the sky. And no matter where I am, I marvel at the wonder of God's creation. Whether I'm looking at the tall palm trees waving in the breeze or the barren, snow-covered branches of East Coast trees stripped of their foliage for the winter, I feel as if I'm in the middle of energy and life, and I'm revitalized. I often use this time to look up to God and say, "How am I doing?" And I try to center myself on the path that I should go.

Whether or not you are as philosophically inclined as I am, walking will provide you with a total-body workout—and without stress on your bones and joints. You'll work your lower body—calves, thighs, hips/buttocks, and abdominals—and your upper body—back, chest, shoulders, and arms. And you'll never feel as if you've strained yourself.

Additional Ways to Burn Fat

SPORTS

One of the most painless ways to burn additional fat is engaging in a favorite sport. You become absorbed in the competition of the game (either with yourself or your partner) and before you know it, you've worked out for an hour or more. But there's one important thing to remember when it comes to using a sport as a part of your fitness regimen: Sports cannot reshape your body and they are rarely equivalent to an aerobic workout. Why?

When you perform a sport, you exercise a particular body part in a certain manner, as is required by the sport. For example, golfers exercise their shoulders and arms, but only at one or two angles. In fact, even though golfers do a lot of shoulder-arm work, I've never seen one who, unless he or she also works out with weights, has beautifully shaped shoulders or arms. The same holds true in any sport. Tennis players have one developed forearm, swimmers have broad backs, and soccer players have developed thighs and calves. But yet even these body parts are not developed and shaped to the best form. Other body parts are completely neglected.

But what about the aerobic effect of sports? Since a sport is rarely done at a continual pace (there are too many stop-and-goes), sports are not usually considered to be strictly aerobic. In addition, most people do not engage in their sport three or more times a week, the recommended amount of aerobic sessions for additional fat burning.

So then, what part do sports play in your fat-burning life? If you enjoy sports, then they should play a major role. I want you to pick a sport or two or even more, and play it as much as your schedule allows. The more you play, the more fat you will burn. However, don't fool yourself into believing that your sport is all that is required to be in shape.

For your information, here is a chart that shows approximately how many calories are burned after playing certain sports for one hour. This, of course, assumes that no breaks are taken.

Sport	Calories Burned per 60 Minutes
Walleyball	600
Racquetball	600
Handball	600
Squash	600
In-line skating	600
Basketball	570
Waterskiing	540
Downhill skiing	540
Rowing	540
Canoeing	540
Roller-skating	540

Sport	Calories Burned per 60 Minutes
Ice-skating	540
Tennis (singles)	480
Tennis (doubles)	420
Volleyball	420
Frisbee	420
Golf	315
Tai chi	300
Yoga	270

Keep in mind that the sport or activity must be done vigorously and nonstop in order to burn the amount of calories in the chart. If you're half asleep, don't expect to reap the same benefit. In other words, if you're anything like me in volleyball and duck every time the ball comes near you, face it, you're not really even in the game! Also note that the chart is a generalization for people of medium height and weight. If you are a big person you will burn more calories than above. If you are a very small person, you may burn a little less than the chart above, but you can compensate for that by putting more energy into your movements.

When it comes to your sport, a general rule is, If you want to burn maximum fat, the goal is to keep on the move and to put everything you have into your moves! In other words, don't stand around in a relaxed manner, even when waiting for the ball. Your body should be tensed from start to finish. Every muscle in your body should be flexed and on the alert. If this ruins the joy of your sport, don't force it. You'll still burn some fat if you play just for enjoyment, but not as much as you would otherwise.

HOUSEHOLD ACTIVITIES

You can burn more fat vacuuming the house than you can sitting on the couch and watching TV! With this in mind, perhaps you can motivate yourself to clean the house more often. For example, if you sit and watch TV for a half an hour, you burn about fifty calories. If you vacuum the house, on the other hand, for the same amount of time, you burn about 105 calories. (Why do you burn any calories sitting and watching TV? Remember, we burn calories twenty-four hours a day—even while sleeping. Breathing itself requires the expenditure of energy. It takes about 2/3 of a calorie to one calorie a minute just to breathe as you sleep!)

But what if you're lazy and just the thought of spending a half hour cleaning or doing other work around the house makes you want to go to the refrigerator and eat? Then just do the chore for ten minutes. You'll still burn some fat. Here is a chart of common household chores and the fat you will burn in ten minutes of work.

Household Activity	Calories Burned Per 10 Minutes
Shoveling snow	125
Washing the walls	100
Painting the walls	90
Washing the car	90
Mowing the lawn	85
Washing the dog	65
Trimming the hedges	50
Weeding the garden	48
Cleaning the windows	40
Mopping the floor	38
Polishing the furniture	38
Vacuuming	35
Raking	35
Dusting	30

DURING THE DAY AT HOME OR OFFICE

You can also burn additional calories during a normal given day. Whether you are at home or in the office, try to do following:

1. Never sit still for more than one hour. If you find yourself sitting at the kitchen table, on the couch, or at a desk, get up and walk around. If possible, stay on your feet five to ten minutes before you sit again.

2. Take a ten-minute walk after each meal! You don't have to do it the moment you finish eating, but within fifteen minutes of the end of your meal, begin your walk. You don't have to walk at a brisk pace. Walk at a leisurely tempo and enjoy yourself, but get moving for that ten minutes. It makes a difference. You'll have to think ahead if you're going to do this at your lunch break at work—and allow the time. Instead of sitting down for the entire hour, get up ten minutes earlier and walk! If you're home and have young children who can't be left, then walk around the house for ten minutes or ride the stationary exercise bike.

3. When talking on the telephone, stand half the time you would ordinarily sit. In other words, if you are used to sitting for ten minutes while talking to your mother on the telephone, sit the

first five minutes and then stand up. After another five minutes, you can sit again. Does this sound crazy? In a way it is, but then so is the whole business of keeping fat off your body in the sedentary world we live in.

4. If you live in an apartment building or work in an office where there are stairs and you feel it is safe, take the stairs rather than the elevator. If you take the subway or bus to work and if your job requires that you sit all day, refuse a seat and stand. Also, when taking the subway, never use the escalator. Take the stairs.

5. When parking your car in a mall, etc., instead of driving around for ten minutes looking for the spot closest to your destination, take a spot that has fewer cars (you may even avoid a fender-bender) and walk the extra distance.

6. In general, remember: It's better to move than be stagnant. It's better to sit up and watch TV than to lie down. It's better to stand up and talk on the telephone than to sit. It's better to walk around the room while talking on the phone than to stand still. It's better to walk quickly from one part of the house to another than to drag along.

7. Remember, in order to burn up one pound of fat, you must use up 3,500 calories. The more active you are, the more calories you burn. Instead of using this information to torture yourself, try to precondition yourself to think action rather than stagnation. Then you'll find yourself automatically choosing the movement mode rather than the vegetation mode. In time it will pay off and you won't think you had to suffer for it.

8. Take your dog on an *extra* walk each day.

But new habits must be established before they become automatic and comfortable. In the beginning you'll be self-conscious about forcing yourself to be more active, and you may resent it. Realize that this too shall pass, and before you know it, you'll be a more energetic person, and it will be more natural for you to move than to be still! Soon people will ask you, "Where do you get all that energy?"

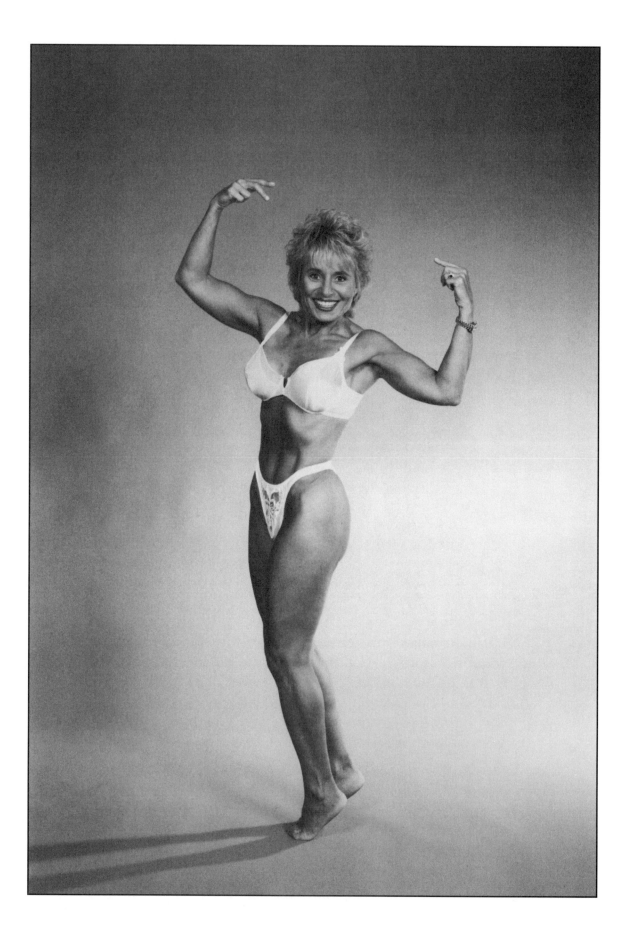

COSMETIC SURGERY AND FAT

If it were possible to get your body in shape with cosmetic surgery, every wealthy woman in the world would have the most beautiful figure possible. Think about it for a moment! Cosmetic surgery is obviously available, and the only thing stopping a person (short of the normal fear of any surgery) is money. With that out of the way, why not do it?

The truth is that many women do it—and not just those with money to spare. Many women go so far as to go into debt in order to get cosmetic surgery in the hope of finally having the body of their dreams. But instead of ending up with the body of their dreams, most of these women are sadly disappointed. There's just no way around it: In order to have a tight, toned, defined, beautifully shaped body at any age, you must work out a certain way. What you've learned in this book so far, and what you will learn in Chapter 10, will give you that body. Cosmetic surgery alone simply can't do it!

What? Am I saying that I am 100 percent against all cosmetic surgery when it comes to the body? No. I am saying that even with cosmetic surgery, you will still have to work out (as all reputable cosmetic surgeons will agree) if you want to be tight and toned—to have firm, defined muscles and to have a beautiful, shapely body. If this is the case, then who should get cosmetic surgery for the body? In my view, very few people. In the following paragraphs you'll find out who they are.

First we'll talk about the most popular form of body cosmetic surgery: liposuction. Then we'll discuss tummy tucks and all sorts of "lifts." In the end you will know what cosmetic surgery can and cannot do for your body.

One more thing. I must say that I am absolutely not against cosmetic surgery for the face, eyes, chin, and neck. Contrary to what you may have heard, these areas cannot be improved by exercise, and must be treated by surgery.

From time to time I get letters from readers asking me if facial and neck exercises can make them look younger. My answer is always no. In fact, the way I see it, facial and neck exercise can cause more lines on the face and neck! How so? When you exercise you not only get muscle, but you get "definition." And what is definition if it is not lines or delineation? The last thing you want on your face, neck, or chin are lines of delineation. And as for muscles on the face, neck, or chin, thankfully, it is very difficult to build them. I say thankfully because if you did build your facial muscles with exercise, you would have a chipmunk-looking face, a wrestler's thick neck, and a hulky, muscular double chin!

The same would go for eyes and brow. You could exercise these areas from now until next New Year's and, at best, nothing would happen. At worst, you would get "definition" or, to put it another way, more lines around your eyes and brow. The truth is that when it comes to the neck and above, unless you want to let those areas age gently with time, the cosmetic surgeon is your best bet. As for me, when the time comes, I shall visit the cosmetic surgeon for facial work without hesitation and age gently with time—only a little more slowly than I would otherwise.

Liposuction: Fat Removal from the Hips, Buttocks, Thighs, or Abdominal Area

Liposuction has been billed as the magic formula for getting rid of excess body fat! The technical terms for this procedure are *suction lipectomy* or *suction-assisted lipectomy*. It is an operation that permanently removes fat cells from specific areas of the body by sucking them out with small tubes. Depending upon how much fat is to be removed and how many areas are involved, the operation can take up to two hours. It is done most safely with an overnight stay in a hospital, and most comfortably, and safely, in my opinion, under general anesthesia. However, it can be done under local anesthesia with sedation in a doctor's office if only a very small area is to be suctioned.

Complete recovery takes about two weeks, although most doctors will suggest that you wait at least three weeks before you start to exercise.

HOW IT IS PERFORMED

The operation is performed by making tiny incisions (about an inch long) in the areas to be suctioned. A small tube is placed in the incision area and moved around in a back-and-forth motion to loosen the fat. The fat is then vacuumed out through the tube. The procedure is made easier and less painful by the injection of large volumes of cold saline water into the fatty tissue. (The water distends the area, making the fat suction more easily and more quickly.)

DO YOU REALLY NEED IT?

Cosmetic surgeons claim that the advantage of liposuction is that it removes a bulge of fat that stubbornly refuses to diminish, even after diet and exercise. But the question is, What kind of dieting and exercise has the potential liposuction patient done before she gives up? My experience with women who were about to get liposuction for thighs, hips, buttocks, and/or stomach tells me that, nine times out of ten—or more—while they may have dieted themselves down to the low-fat ideal body weight, they did not do the proper exercises. Most of them have tried endless aerobics and/or lengthy abdominal and/or hips-butt-thighs classes where they do a series of exercises for these body parts that are not the most effective way to sculpt the body.

When I encourage these women to work out in the way described in this and my other books, they come back in six months to a year and tell me, "I never would have believed it. I was about to get liposuction and now my thighs are firm and defined—and most of the cellulite is gone," or "My stomach is finally getting tight and toned—and I see definition all over. I'm going to keep doing your workout instead of getting surgery," or "Thank God I didn't get liposuction on my buttocks. All I needed was your hips/butt and thigh workout." (Some thigh exercises also lift and shape the buttocks.)

Am I saying that liposuction is an unnecessary operation, period, and in every case it can be eliminated by diet and exercise? No. The truth is that, while in most cases if you follow my workout plan to a T, in time your body will look better than it would had you had liposuction and not exercised, there are certain cases where, after all is said and done, there will still be a small, annoying pocket of fat that stubbornly remains. But even in such cases, often it is only because the person needs to lose those last few pounds of fat.

For example, if I didn't know better, I would think that I needed liposuction on my lower stomach. Why? In spite of all my exercise, when I am even a pound or two overweight, my lower belly protrudes!

However, when I diet down and get rid of that last pound of excess fat, my lower belly is absolutely flat. So I would never get liposuction.

WHAT LIPOSUCTION CAN AND CANNOT DO

But what if even after you've done the workout as prescribed in my books and dieted down to that last pound of excess fat, you still have a pocket or two of unsightly fat on your body? Should you get liposuction or should you just live with it? The choice is yours. I would live with it. But if you do decide upon liposuction, remember one thing: Liposuction cannot make your body firm, nor can it give you definition. You must still work out in order to do that. (Only muscle makes the body firm and defined. Liposuction simply removes fat. It cannot create muscle.)

THE IDEAL TIME TO GET LIPOSUCTION

For optimum results, you must get it when you are already dieted down to your ideal weight. Why? The operation is limited to the amount of tissue that can be removed at one time safely. (Fat cells do not multiply when you gain weight; they merely get bigger.) When you are at your thinnest, your fat cells are at their smallest in size and the surgeon can remove the greatest number of cells. (If, on the other hand, you were at your fattest, your fat cells would be larger in size and the surgeon would only be able to remove a certain amount of tissue safely and would be forced to leave behind many fat cells. This would mean that you would remain partially fat, or need another operation.)

WHEN YOU GAIN A FEW POUNDS THE FAT HAS TO GO SOMEWHERE!

There's a big problem when it comes to getting liposuction. If you gain weight at any time in your life, even a few pounds (and if you are human, trust me, you will), since the fat can never return to the area from which the fat cells were removed, it must go somewhere else—and you never know where it will go. Let me explain.

Suppose you had liposuction on your butt. Years ago, before I started working out, I was thinking of getting my butt made smaller by liposuction. But then I read that the fat cells would go somewhere else if I gained weight. I already knew that my last bit of fat tends to go to my lower stomach. I pictured yet more fat landing on that area—and I envisioned myself looking pregnant twelve months of the year. So I decided not to do it. Later, after working out, my butt was lifted and shaped by the workout and I'm delighted with it.

You could think positive and believe that if you gain weight, the fat will go where you want it to go—for example, to your breasts and nowhere else. But while this could happen, it's as likely as winning the lottery. You could think another way and say, "Okay. I'll beat the system. I'll have liposuction on my butt, my hips, my thighs, and my stomach. This way the fat can never return to any of those areas." Fine. But as mentioned above, if you gain weight, you will store excess body fat somewhere. The fat may go to your neck, your ankles, your knees, or it may form itself in a jelly roll around your lower back. In any case, it *will* appear and, chances are, in a most inconvenient place. You may find yourself wishing that you'd never had the liposuction; at least this way, when you gained weight, you would not have to worry about looking misshapen.

Don't mind me. I'm a pessimist when it comes to cosmetic surgery to shape the body! I'm sure you could have a positive experience. But I do want you to keep in mind the very real issues when it comes to this decision.

WHAT ABOUT CELLULITE?

Finally, can liposuction remove cellulite? Until recently, no! When the excess fat was removed by liposuction, the craterlike appearance of the skin remained. However, some cosmetic surgeons claim that recent advances in the process of fat removal now allow the surgeon to break the fibrous bridges that cause the dimpled look of cellulite. Not every cosmetic surgeon is aware of this procedure, however. It was discovered by Brazilian and Italian surgeons.

Once again, I must emphasize that by proper diet and correct working out, you can get rid of most, if not all, of your cellulite. As you diet, the fat diminishes. As you work out, you create a muscle under the skin. In time, this muscle creates a smooth area and the skin over it is no longer dimpled and craterlike. (See pp. 3–4 for a review of this subject.)

One more point. Depending upon how much fat you've had removed, the body part that had liposuction may sag down and need further surgery, a "lift," to get rid of the excess skin. For example, you may need a tummy tuck, a mini tummy tuck, a thigh or butt lift, and so on. A competent surgeon will help you to avoid this problem by giving you an accurate evaluation in the first place so that you can get what is needed done at the same time and not have to go back for further surgery.

BEWARE: YOUR SKIN CAN BECOME DISCOLORED

Even if you have the best surgeon available anywhere, you may have permanent skin discoloration in the areas where you've had liposuction. In other words, you may have patches of blotchy brown coloration on your stomach, hips, buttocks, thighs—anywhere where fat was sucked from your skin. Your doctor will speak to you to find out what your odds are of having this problem; however, he or she cannot tell for sure. It is always a risk.

Full and Mini Tummy Tucks

A full tummy tuck is the most drastic surgery discussed in this chapter. The technical name for it is *abdominal lipectomy with repair of diastasis recti, resection of lipocutaneous excess, and repair of umbilical or abdominal hernia*. The operation involves the removal of excess body fat around the entire upper and lower abdominal area, the sewing up of loose muscle to tighten that area, the removal of excess skin, and the necessary repositioning of the navel. The operation takes two to three hours and is always performed in a hospital. It usually requires a two-to-three-day stay in the hospital.

The healing process is about four to six weeks. You should wait at least six to eight weeks before you resume your full exercise program.

HOW IT IS PERFORMED

The operation is performed by first removing the excess fat around the entire abdominal area, just as is done by liposuction described above. Next, the deep layer of fat is separated from the abdominal muscle, from the top of the muscle down to the navel. The skin is then freed from the navel and the surrounding area, all the way to the ribs. Now, with a clear field to work on the abdominal muscles, the surgeon pulls the stretched muscle together by stitching it down the middle from the ribs to the pubic bone. After that, excess skin is pulled tight and removed.

You will have a scar in the lower abdominal area that may remain lumpy, firm, and red for up to eighteen months. The scar is in the best possible of places, just above the pubic bone and running across to either side of your body. Even in a skimpy bikini, no one would see it!

DO YOU REALLY NEED IT?

In my opinion, women who may need this operation are those who, through many pregnancies, have damaged muscles to the point where they are unable to respond to exercise. You will know whether or not this applies to you if you have dieted down to your proper weight and, in addition, have done the workout in this book or that found in *Gut Busters* or in my *Bottoms Up Workout: Middle Body* video for one year, with little or no results. (Chances of this happening are very slim—98 percent of the women who've written to me thinking that they fall into this category find out to their delight that after working out for a year, they see major improvement and opt to keep going with the exercise.)

WHAT A FULL TUMMY TUCK CAN AND CANNOT DO

A full tummy tuck can remove vast amounts of excess fat from your entire abdominal area and flatten that area to some extent, but it cannot give you a completely flat abdominal area, nor can it give you definition. Don't even dream that a tummy tuck can give you "washboard abs." For that you will have to do exercises after your stomach heals enough so that you can exercise. (Note that all surgeons agree that in order to obtain a firm, defined stomach, it is also necessary to begin a regular exercise regimen for the stomach and to continue that regimen for life!)

THE IDEAL TIME TO GET A FULL TUMMY TUCK

If you are going to get a tummy tuck, it's most important that you wait until you are finished with pregnancies. Otherwise, your repaired muscles may stretch again and you'll have to undergo more surgery. In addition, it's important that you try to shape up your stomach muscles as much as possible before the operation. If you do this, you will heal in less time than you would otherwise heal and will be able to exercise more quickly after surgery.

BEWARE: IF YOU GET REALLY FAT, YOU COULD AGAIN STRETCH OUT YOUR MUSCLES

We've already discussed what may happen if you get pregnant again after a tummy tuck, but gaining a lot of weight (fifty or more pounds) can be just as damaging. You can stretch out your muscles once again and have to go through the surgery all over. The truth is, if you're not planning to go into a lifetime diet and exercise program, it's not a good idea to get a tummy tuck.

MINI TUMMY TUCK

A mini tummy tuck is much less drastic than a full tummy tuck. In essence, it is a tummy tuck for the area below the waistline only. The technical name for it is *modified abdominal sipectom with repair of inferior diastasis rectus and resection of lipocutaneous excess*. In this operation, excess fat is removed from the lower abdominal area, the lower abdominal muscles are sewn and tightened, and excess skin is removed.

The operation takes one to two hours and, in my opinion, it should always be done with at least an overnight stay in a hospital and under general anesthesia, although some doctors will perform it in an office using local sedation. It takes about four to six weeks before you can return to your normal activities.

HOW IT IS PERFORMED

The fat is suctioned from your lower stomach area in the same way as is done with liposuction. The rest of the operation follows the same procedures as a full tummy tuck, only instead of pulling the skin away from both the upper and lower abdominal area, sewing up the entire abdominal muscle, and cutting a volume of skin, the surgeon works only on the lower abdominal area, and there is less trauma to the body. The result is a much smaller scarring area; however, just as in a regular tummy tuck, your scarred area may remain lumpy, firm, and red for up to eighteen months. The scar runs horizontally across the pubic bone area. The navel is not moved in this operation.

DO YOU REALLY NEED IT?

If your lower stomach protrudes no matter how much exercise you do—and if you've followed this workout, *Gut Busters*, or *The Bottoms Up Workout: Middle Body* video for a year—and have dieted down to your ideal weight and if you have a small pot on your lower belly along with a pocket of skin sagging above your pubic bone, you may want to consider this operation. Frankly, I've encouraged many women to take up my challenge and give it a year of following my workout. The result is that the only women who ended up getting surgery were those who told me flat out that they didn't have the patience to wait a year to see what would happen. Since they had the money and the inclination, they decided that they would get the operation and then do the workout.

WHAT A MINI TUMMY TUCK CAN AND CANNOT DO

This operation will give you a somewhat flatter, tighter lower abdominal area. It will in no way affect your upper abdominals. However, the operation will not give you a lower abdominal area that is flat as a board, nor will it produce defined muscle. It only tightens your existing muscle.

THE IDEAL TIME TO GET A MINI TUMMY TUCK

As with a full tummy tuck, you should wait until you are finished with pregnancies before undergoing this operation, otherwise your repaired muscles and tucked skin may stretch again, and you'll have to get more surgery. Also as with the full tummy tuck, be sure that you don't gain a great deal of weight again—or your hard-earned money and investment of precious time and energy in this operation may be wasted.

Hip, Thigh, and Butt Lifts

The technical term for this operation is *resection of lipocutaneous excess of hips, thighs, and buttocks*, or *body contouring of hips, thighs, and buttocks*. The operation is designed to tighten loose and/or "hanging" skin on these areas. The operation is always done in a hospital (the stay is one to two nights) under general anesthesia.

Complete recovery takes about two weeks, although most doctors will suggest that you wait three to four weeks before you resume a full exercise program.

HOW IT IS PERFORMED

The body part being "lifted" has been premarked either the night before or an hour before surgery. The surgeon then makes incisions in the marked areas and injects a dilute epinephrine (adrenaline) into them to limit excessive bleeding. Then, following the markings, the surgeon removes the excess skin down to the muscle and, along with it, usually a thick layer of fat under the skin. If it is your thigh that is being lifted, your thigh skin is raised as high as possible on your leg. The excess skin is later cut off and the wound is sewn up. The same is done for the buttocks or hips: Excess skin is pulled down or aside, and later cut off and the wound sewn up.

DO YOU REALLY NEED IT?

The "lift" type of cosmetic surgery on the hips, thighs, and butt is in my opinion, the least necessary cosmetic surgery available. Working out, particularly with weights, is a far more effective remedy to sagging flesh than any cosmetic surgery.

I have never seen a woman using one of my exercise routines who has not been able to lift her thighs, hips, or buttocks. If you have thighs that sag significantly, you may have to use heavier weights than the five-pound dumbbells suggested in this book. In fact, you may want to switch to my book *Now or Never*, or *Top Shape*, at least for thigh work—and use a barbell and a squat rack for heavier thigh work. If you do this, in time, not only will you have performed a wonderful thigh lift (without any stitches), but your thighs will gain a beautiful shape that no surgical process could ever duplicate. It will take six months to a year to complete this "operation."

The same holds true for the hips and buttocks, and in fact, it is the same exercises—squats and lunges done with heavy weights—that lift the skin on the hips/buttocks area. So if your thighs, hips, or buttocks have hanging skin and you find that the *Bathing Suit Workout* or the workouts with lighter weights don't do it, go to *Now or Never* and follow the heavy-duty thigh workout there—with the goal of gradually building up to the heavier weights—and you will solve your problem.

Am I saying that thigh, hip, and butt lifts are never needed? No. In cases where medical reasons prevent an individual from working out with weights, then the surgery is the only way to lift the sagging skin. But in such cases you must realize that you cannot hope to get the same results you would get through working out.

WHAT HIP, BUTTOCK, AND THIGH LIFTS CAN AND CANNOT DO

As described above, surgical "lifts" can raise sagging skin so that it no longer hangs down in an unsightly manner. However, lifts can never make your body feel firm, nor can lifts give the lifted body part a pretty shape or definition. After all, lifts do not create muscles. In order to re-shape your thighs, hips, or buttocks, for example, the surgeon would have to use muscle implants. There has been some experimentation in these areas, but little success. And in any case, if they do perfect a way to implant muscle all over the body, we could be walking around with our own skeletons and a whole body of artificial muscle. I don't think the human body would stand for such a thing, do you? So I guess we'd better resign ourselves to shaping our bodies the way Nature intended—by exercising them, making muscles naturally—and keeping ourselves strong and healthy.

BEWARE: YOU MAY BE DISAPPOINTED

If you got your hip, butt, or thigh lift in the hope of showing off your new, "tight" body part, you may be sadly disappointed if you're not lucky when it comes to scarring. Even if your doctor is highly skilled in making sure that your scars are placed in the least noticeable areas, your scars can widen or shift. In addition, should you get an infection while in the healing process, the scars could become permanently lumpy. Can you imagine yourself wearing a bathing suit with ribbonlike scars under your buttocks and on your upper thighs? Not everyone will have this problem, but it's something to think about.

Making the Decision: To Do or Not to Do

Before you make the decision to get cosmetic surgery on your body, ask yourself the following questions and answer them honestly:

1. Does my medical doctor agree that I am physically incapable of working out with weights as described in my workout book? If he or she does not agree and says that you should try exercise, then:

2. Have I tried the workout for this body part for at least a year? If so, have I followed the workout exactly as written? Have I gradually raised my weights in order to create a muscle that would lift the skin? If you are still not satisfied with the results, then:

3. Is it important enough for me to spend the money that will be required for the operation? If you think it is, then ask yourself:

4. Am I willing to take the risks involved with the operation (scarring, discoloration, fat going to other places, future sagging if excessive weight is regained and then lost again, etc.)?

If after all of the above thinking you still want to get cosmetic surgery on your body, it is your choice. You have every right to do what you want to do. After all, it's your money, your body, and your life. No one should make your decisions for you.

Finding a Reputable Cosmetic Surgeon

First, if you are seriously thinking of cosmetic surgery, I suggest that you read the book *The Complete Book of Cosmetic Surgery*, or another complete guide to the cosmetic surgery of your choosing. Such a book will give you a much more detailed understanding of what is involved in the operation you are considering. It will also give more particulars than I will give here on how to find a competent surgeon to perform the operation.

In the following paragraphs, I'll offer a brief outline of the "musts" to keep in mind before agreeing to an operation with a given doctor.

As shocking as it may seem, any doctor, as long as he or she is licensed by a given state to practice medicine, can call him- or herself a "cosmetic," or "plastic," surgeon. This doctor may have a general degree with no specialization in cosmetic surgery. For this reason, you must be sure that the doctor you choose is "board certified." But board certified by whom? The surgeon must be certified by a board approved by the American Academy of Facial Plastic and Reconstructive Surgery. If the doctor has such certification, you can be sure that he or she has spent many years studying and practicing specifically in the field of cosmetic surgery—and is not just a general doctor who happens to think he or she is talented in cosmetic surgery.

One of the best ways to find a cosmetic surgeon is by recommendation of someone who has had success with that surgeon. If you are lucky enough to know such a person, however, don't forget to ask the doctor if he or she is board certified as above—and, in fact, to ask to see his or her certification, which should certainly be hanging on the wall, prominently displayed.

If you really want to be sure of your surgeon's history, ask to see what is called his or her curriculum vitae. It will give a full report on his or her schooling, medical practice experience, etc. You can then count the years he or she has spent specifically studying cosmetic surgery, as well as the years he or she has spent practicing his or her art. (And cosmetic surgery is indeed an art! The way I see it, this doctor is really an artist, sculpting your face or body. In fact, I think talent, as well as skill, is needed.)

If you don't know where to find a doctor, call your county medical society. They will be happy to supply a list of qualified, board-certified surgeons in the area where you are considering surgery.

Another way to go is to get hold of a copy of *The Directory of Medical Specialists*, which is available at most libraries or on the Internet. It lists all board-certified surgeons according to their specialties and the area where they live. The book comes in a few volumes and can be intimidating. If you have trouble, don't hesitate to ask your librarian to help you. Librarians are wonderful people who delight in doing just that!

A Final Word about Cosmetic Surgery on the Body

Cosmetic surgery can lift skin and cut away the excess. It can suck out the fat cells from a given area. It can even, in some cases, sew together a loose muscle, tightening that muscle. But cosmetic surgery can never create muscles on your body, and it can never make you physically stronger. Only exercise can do that. Finally, cosmetic surgery cannot sculpt and shape your muscles into their most perfect form. So even if you do get cosmetic surgery, plan on working out. There's simply no substitute.

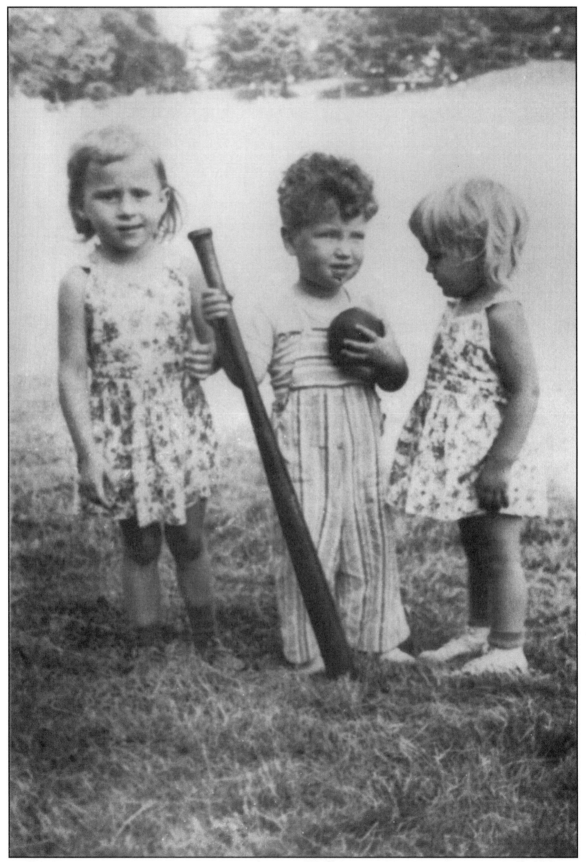

Joyce Vedral—the little chunky one—getting ready to snatch the ball!

10

KEEP IT OFF! THIS MEANS THE FLAB!

You've taken the first step. You're in shape. What? How dare I say that getting in shape is only "the first step" after all the work you've done? Haven't you taken all the steps you need to take? No. *Getting in shape is only the initial step to a beautiful, fit, low-fat body for the rest of your life.* Steps two, three, four, five, and all the way to infinity are to follow as you heed the advice in this chapter.

In the following paragraphs, you will learn not only how to keep the beautiful body you have achieved, but also how to improve on that body. You'll discover ways to sculpt your physique so that not only your hips/butt, thigh, and abdominal areas look great, but your other body parts as well: chest, shoulders, back, biceps, triceps, and calves. But your goal will be not only to work out in order to get the rest of your body looking beautiful. It will also be to add muscle to your overall body, muscle that will create for you a fat-burning furnace that allows you to eat more without putting on weight. And don't worry. I'm not talking about hulking, masculine muscles. I'm referring to the petite, sexy, shapely muscles that give the body its best form. And speaking of form, look at my form at two years old! I'm the one eyeing the ball.

In addition, you'll want to work with weights so that you have an insurance policy against future bone thinning (osteoporosis). As mentioned in Chapter 7, my bones are almost double the density of women my age—and more dense than in-shape twenty-five-year-olds. So let's get started. First we'll talk about diet and then we'll discuss how to incorporate this workout with other weight-training workouts or how to switch to a different workout completely—for the sake of variety, for a lifetime of fitness.

Diet: Maintaining Your Low-Fat Body

Thankfully, as discussed in Chapter 7, once you've eliminated your excess body fat and like what you see in the mirror, you can eat anything you want once a week. But what if, for some reason, you throw all caution to the wind and eat what you will for months at a time—and find yourself carrying five, ten, or more pounds of fat on your body?

All is not lost. In fact, you are better off than you were when you started. At least now you have learned that gaining and losing body fat is not based upon luck and chance but is instead a very reliable science. Just as surely as the tide comes in and goes out again, when you eat more calories than you burn, you add body fat. When you burn more calories than you eat, you lose body fat. It's an immutable law of nature. It won't change no matter what you do.

It's an Emotional Issue

For most of us, weight gain is an emotional issue. When we cannot zip up our jeans, or when that form-fitting dress rides up around our hips, we don't just logically say to ourselves, "Oh well. I've eaten more calories than I've burned and I've stored some fat. I guess I'll have to reverse the process and start losing the stored fat." Instead we panic and imagine that not only will we never get rid of the fat, but we will continue to get fatter and fatter, no matter what we do.

We also imagine that no matter what we do the fat will never come off! It is our guilt that makes us feel this way. We condemn ourselves for not having been more alert, blame ourselves for not exercising more self-control. Instead of acknowledging the fact that overeating is both normal and human, we become angry with ourselves. We look at ourselves in repulsion and hatred. "You're disgusting," we think. "You have neither self-discipline nor self-respect," we accuse. These feelings and thoughts depress us. And when we feel depressed, we try to make ourselves feel better by—you guessed it—eating more.

Break the Cycle by Changing Your Thinking!

It's a vicious circle. But it can be stopped by changing our thought process, by getting back to logic and not psychological voodoo that dooms us to failure. Gaining weight is based upon very predictable laws of science.

Think about it. If you fill a glass beyond its capacity, the water flows over the rim. There is no chance that one day things are going to change and suddenly when you fill a glass beyond its capacity, the water is going to start piling itself up in the air. Ridiculous! Right? The same way, when you sip away at a drink of water, the water level goes down and down. As you use up the water, there is less in the glass. There is no way that one day while you're sipping a glass of water, you will suddenly be able to sip away forever and the water level will not go down and the water will eventually not be consumed.

So it is with excess body fat. There are scientific, unchanging laws that apply. You gained the weight according to the laws of nature, and you will lose the weight the same way. Don't panic. Talk to yourself. Realize that just as you gained the excess fat, slowly, consistently, over time, you will lose it. Go back to the eating plan in Chapter 7 until you reach your goal, then once again you can eat anything you want once a week. And if you've stopped working out, start up again. Which brings me to my next point.

Never Stop Working Out!

When it comes to working out, people ask me, "Will I have to do this for the rest of my life?" They say it as if they're being condemned to lifetime imprisonment. Their attitude is all wrong. Dreading exercise is like dreading getting out of bed every day. Regardless of how much you like to sleep, you've already resigned yourself to that necessity. If you remained in bed forever, you would get bedsores, your muscles would atrophy, your bones would thin. Your entire body would eventually deteriorate. The same attitude should apply to exercise.

Of course you must do it every day—or at least almost every day. Why? Most of us don't do enough exercise naturally and we need a regular exercise regimen to make up for that. We must incorporate a workout regimen into our daily life. So instead of looking at exercise as a life sentence, think of it as necessary maintenance—like brushing your teeth, taking a shower, and even eating.

It Doesn't Have to Be Boring

Even though your exercise regimens will become as natural as your daily hygienic routines, thankfully you can incorporate more variety into them than you can into brushing your teeth or taking a shower! (There are only so many ways to brush your teeth, and only so many varieties of bath and shower soaps, oils, perfumes, and sponges you can try.)

In the following paragraphs you'll find various workouts that you can switch to from time to time, for the rest of your life, so that you can stay in top shape and at the same time never be bored with your workout. But first I must point out that no matter which routines you decide to follow, it's important that eventually you add exercises for the body parts that are not working in your Bathing Suit Workout—otherwise your middle body will look tight, toned, sexy, and defined, but your upper body will look sad in contrast.

Adding the Rest of the Body Parts to Your Bathing Suit Workout

It's easy to make your workout complete. Just select one of the books listed below and add in the body parts you are not exercising in the Bathing Suit Workout, leaving out the hips/buttocks, thigh, and abdominal workout for that routine and continuing to do your Bathing Suit Workout for those body parts. Later, when you get bored with the Bathing Suit Workout, you can stop doing that routine and do any of the total-body workouts (they are all total-body workouts) listed below. Then later, if you choose, you can again go back to the Bathing Suit Workout and continue doing the rest of your body parts with one of the routines in this chapter.

The closest system to your Bathing Suit routine, and the one that will net you the highest muscle quality for your time investment, is the upper-body workout in the book *Bottoms Up!*, or *Definition* or *The Fat-Burning Workout.*

Both of these routines employ the method of the superset or "twin set." It is exactly the same method as you use in *The Bathing Suit Workout*, except instead of exercising three different body parts before you take a rest, you exercise only two body parts. For example, in *Bottoms Up!*, you do one set of chest exercises and one set of shoulder exercises. Then you take a fifteen-second rest and repeat the sequence until you have finished those two exercises. You then move to the next two exercises for chest and shoulders, and so on, until you have completed your entire chest-shoulder routine. You then move to the next combination, arms—and you "twin-set" biceps and triceps. Finally, you combine back and calves (yes, the one lower body part that makes me a liar! You are not really working only upper body, but calves were left out of your Bathing Suit Workout, and they are paired with the back in *Bottoms Up!*).

If you are doing the Bathing Suit Workout, you will of course leave out the lower- and middle-body routine of *Bottoms Up!* It is an excellent routine and a welcome change to your Bathing Suit Workout, and after, say, three months, you may want to switch completely to that workout. But for now, simply add in the six missing body parts as mentioned above: chest/shoulders, biceps/triceps, and back and calves.

If you choose to do the workout in *Definition*, you will be using the same method—supersetting—but within the same body part, and your combinations will be different, and some of the exercises will also be different. In addition, instead of doing three sets per body part, you'll be doing five. If you choose to do the Fat-Burning Workout, you'll be doing the giant set but with different exercises and different combinations. Review Chapter 2 and see which workouts the before-and-after women did for the upper body.

I advise you to pick one or the other immediately and add it to your Bathing Suit routine. Along with your Bathing Suit routine, do that for three to six months. Then stop doing your Bathing Suit routine and do the total body workout in that book. If you want an intense workout for your hips/buttocks, thigh, and abdominal areas, do the entire workout in *Bottoms Up!* If you want a less intense but yet very effective workout for those areas, do the entire workout found in workout level 4 of *Weight Training Made Easy*, or use my book *Definition*.

What to Do as Time Goes By!

Okay. Fine. But what do you do as the years go by? Do you have to keep up that same old routine, doing your Bathing Suit Workout but adding the missing body parts from either of the above books and from time to time stopping the Bathing Suit Workout and doing the entire workout from one of the above books? No. Thankfully, you have a choice of many other effective workouts that will not only give you the feeling of variety, but in addition will help to perfect your body still further and provide a workout that will suit your specific life situation. At any time, you can do the Bathing Suit Workout for hips/buttocks, thighs, and abdominals and add in the routines for the missing body parts—chest, shoulders, biceps, triceps, and calves—found in any of the books listed below, or you can stop doing the Bathing Suit Workout and do the total-body workout found in any of the books listed below.

From Shortest to Longest—From Least Muscle to Most Muscle

Except for *Weight Training Made Easy*, which is presented last, the workouts presented below are given in the order of least time consuming to most time consuming—and from the least muscle yielding to the most muscle yielding. For intensity or difficulty, see the particular descriptions. Note that the three specialized workouts are discussed separately.

THE 12-MINUTE TOTAL-BODY WORKOUT

The 12-Minute Total-Body Workout is the least intimidating of all of my workout books. It allows you to become acquainted with exercising the rest of your body with weights without asking you to commit a whole lot of time. All you need is twelve minutes a day.

You need only one set of three-pound dumbbells in order to do the workout and, in fact, since you create your own force by flexing your muscles hard (isometric pressure), you could actually do the workout with no weights. For this reason, it is also ideal for traveling.

Although this workout does not increase muscle size at all unless you have very underdeveloped muscles, it does produce what all women want: firmness or "muscle hardness." And it is so simple to perform that you wonder how it could be so effective.

You exercise each body part individually, doing two exercises for each body part—three sets each. You do ten repetitions for each set. But in order to make up for the fact that you are using very light weights, you must create your own "work" by using "dynamic tension" and "isometric pressure." In other words, you continually put force on the working muscle by flexing and tensing it throughout the movement. Because of the continual flexing and tensing, every muscle fiber participates in each movement—and, in turn, your muscles become more firm.

If you want to begin a total-body workout and you feel a bit intimidated about starting, this would be the ideal place to begin. I do it myself for weeks at a time when I am burned out and feel like having an easier workout. I also use it when I'm on the road and don't have access to weights. As mentioned above, you could either add this to your Bathing Suit Workout, leaving out the hips/buttocks, thighs, and abdominals, or you could stop doing the Bathing Suit Workout for a while and simply do the entire 12-Minute Total-Body Workout.

DEFINITION: SHAPE WITHOUT BULK IN FIFTEEN MINUTES A DAY

Definition does exactly what it says: It gives you paramount definition and muscle shaping without adding much muscle size. You burn maximum fat while working out—and in fact, if you don't take your optional rests, the workout is completely aerobic. You go so fast that you can do it in fifteen minutes a day. What's more, if you choose you can double up with this workout and do your entire body in one day. Your time investment of thirty minutes will allow you to work out only three days a week. Other than *Top Shape*, which allows men to do this only if they are not exercising their legs, it's the only other book I've written that allows only three days of working out.

Use *Definition* if you're looking for a greater challenge than *The 12-Minute Total Body Workout* and you want to burn the utmost amount of fat and get more delineation.

For this workout, you do five sets of each exercise as you utilize the workout principal called the full pyramid system. With this method, you add weight to each of your first three sets, then decrease the weight for your last two sets, until you return to your original weight, for a total of five sets. (This is the only one of my books that utilizes the full pyramid system.) You use three sets of very light dumbbells, perhaps ones, twos, and threes (heavier if you are strong enough). You work in "speed supersets," doing one set each of two different exercises for the same body part and then, without resting, raising your weight and repeating the sequence, and so on, until all five supersets (ten sets in all) have been completed.

Since there are five sets per body part, only two exercises per body part provide a complete and intense workout. However, an optional two exercises per body part are given for those who wish to be Wonder Women or Dragon Ladies.

THE FAT-BURNING WORKOUT

The Fat-Burning Workout takes twenty minutes to do (there are optional "intensity" and "insanity" workouts that add ten minutes each to the workout). This workout allows for more muscle development than *Definition*, yet it still allows you to burn maximum fat. You do the workout by using what is called the giant set. Here, you do one set each of three different exercises for the same body part before taking a fifteen-second rest. You will notice that you did something similar in your Bathing Suit Workout. You did one set each of three different exercises before taking a fifteen-second rest, only you did one set each of three different exercises for three different body parts: hips/buttocks, thighs, and abdominals. In *The Fat-Burning Workout*, you work within the body part. (For example, you would do one set each of three different exercises for thighs before taking a fifteen-second rest.)

This workout utilizes the modified pyramid system. It requires that you go up the pyramid, adding weight to each of your first three sets. Then you stop. By way of contrast, with *Definition*, you were required to do the full pyramid system, where you not only ascend the pyramid but also descend it. (In that workout, you are asked to go down the pyramid, doing two additional sets by decreasing the weight until you return to your original weight.)

The Fat-Burning Workout is less intense than *Definition*. You are allowed to rest after three sets rather than after ten sets! In *Definition*, not only are you using the "true pyramid," which requires that you do five sets before you take a rest, but you are also speed-supersetting two exercises (see above) so with that workout, you are actually doing ten sets before you take a rest.

The Fat-Burning Workout asks you to use three-, five-, and eight-pound dumbbells, but you don't have to go that high. You can start with dumbbells as light as one, two, and three pounds and gradually increase your weights. Also, as with any other of my workouts, over time you can increase your weights still further.

With this workout, you can get more muscle than with either *The 12-Minute Total-Body Workout* or *Definition*—but don't worry, not the bulky kind, but sexy, defined, taut muscle.

If you decide to do this workout, it's very important that you get and read the book first, even though you can also purchase this workout in video! There are many important tips in the book, and the book provides motivational talk.

The video is no longer available in stores, so you can order it by writing to me at my P.O. box. Volume I is a forty-minute video that has only the regular workout. (You will not do forty minutes a day, but twenty minutes for upper body on workout day one, and the other twenty minutes for lower body on workout day two, and so on.) Volume II is an eighty-minute video that has the intensity and insanity workouts. (Again, you will not do an eighty-minute workout in one day, but will divide your workout into days one and two.)

If you have gone past the regular workout, you won't need Volume I—just Volume II. See p. 199 for prices and ordering information.

THE COLLEGE DORM WORKOUT

You don't have to go to college to do it! The College Dorm Workout takes only twenty minutes to do! It is very similar to The Fat-Burning Workout, only even less complicated, and you get slightly less muscle and definition than you do with The Fat-Burning Workout. You never have to raise your weight (you don't use the pyramid system, or even the modified pyramid system). You use one set of five-pound dumbbells for sets of all exercises. What's more, you don't even need an exercise bench. The workout was designed for people with a small workout area. All you need is a chair, the floor, yourself, the dumbbells, and a five-by-six-foot space!

For this workout, you do three exercises for each body part—ten repetitions each. You "giant set," just as in *The Fat-Burning Workout*, doing one set each of three different exercises for a given body part before you take a rest. Only, as stated above, instead of doing your next set with a higher weight, you continue to work with the same weight. But in order to compensate for the lack of added weight, you are asked to squeeze your working muscle as hard as possible throughout the movement, utilizing the principles of "dynamic tension" and "isometric pressure" as is used in *The 12-Minute Total-Body Workout*.

In addition, the book provides handy tips on eating in difficult situations. What is described for college-life eating scenarios—parties, cafeterias with limited offerings, etc.—can be applied to other situations—restaurants, eating dinner at people's homes, etc. Except for *Gut Busters*, the book is smaller, less expensive, and less intimidating than any of my other books.

BOTTOMS UP!

Bottoms Up! takes twenty minutes to do if you don't take your optional rests; otherwise it takes about thirty minutes, unless you choose the optional Wild Woman and Terminator workouts, which add ten minutes each to the workout. This workout allows for more muscle development than any of the above workouts—yet, because you are rarely resting, it allows you to burn maximum fat. (You can't build hulky muscles with this or any of my workouts. I'm talking about firm, sexy muscles here!)

You are able to develop more muscle with this workout because of the way you work out. Instead of bombing away at one body part with multiple sets, you are constantly switching back and forth between two body parts. You are not stopping your workout by taking rests but, on the other hand, you are allowing certain body parts to rest: While one body part is working, another body part is resting. As mentioned above, it is most similar to your Bathing Suit Workout, only here you are exercising two body parts at a time, whereas in the Bathing Suit Workout you exercise three body parts at a time.

This workout requires that you work in twin sets, where you do one set of, say, a hips/buttocks exercise and then, without resting, one set of a thigh exercise, and so on. But *Bottoms Up!* provides a more intense workout for the lower and middle body than for the upper body. Seven twin sets are required for lower, five for middle, and three for upper (although Wild Woman and Terminator options are given, to extend the upper-body challenge).

The workout utilizes the modified pyramid system (the same as is used in *The Fat-Burning Workout*). You gradually increase your weight for the first three sets, using three-, five-, and ten-pound dumbbells. (Of course you can start with lower weights and work your way up, eventually to as high as ten-, fifteen-, and twenty-pound dumbbells.)

Even if you love the Bathing Suit Workout, after a while it's a good idea to switch to the entire *Bottoms Up!* workout, *The Fat-Burning Workout*, or *Definition*. You'll be hitting your hips/buttocks, thighs, and abdominals from different angles and, in time, improving your shape even more—because muscles need a change to be challenged.

In addition to being in book form, this workout is on video on three volumes: *The Bottoms Up Workout: Lower Body*; *The Bottoms Up Workout: Middle Body*; and *The Bottoms Up Workout: Upper Body*. But don't just get the videos. You must first read the book for motivation, the diet, and other important information. You can purchase the videos by writing to me at my P.O. box. See p. 199.

TOP SHAPE

Top Shape is billed as a men's book. In fact, the byline reads, "Now Joyce shows men what to do." Yet the book is a women's workout as well as a man's workout! The reason I addressed the book to men is that there are some things that men do differently than women. First, they don't have to exercise their hips/buttocks area the way we do. They get enough of a butt workout when they do thigh exercises such as squats and lunges. Also, since men can eat more than women and still lose body fat, there is a special diet just for men in this book. Other than that, women can follow the book. This book allows you to build more muscle than any book yet discussed.

Since *Top Shape* is my only book that has a machine workout using a home gym machine (as well as a dumbbell workout, of course), you may find this book very helpful if you have a home gym machine and wish to do the machine substitutes listed in all of my books. In addition, *Top Shape* has a regular dumbbell workout that allows more rests than any of the above workouts—and in this sense it is the least exhausting.

The workout takes thirty minutes and is done four to six days a week. It allows you to rest fifteen seconds after each and every set of exercises. It utilizes the modified pyramid system as is used in *The Fat-Burning Workout* and *Bottoms Up!*, where you add weight to each of three sets. Men begin with three-, five-, and ten-pound dumbbells or higher, depending on their beginning strength, and work their way up to as high as twenty-five, thirty, or thirty-five pounds or higher. Women begin at the same weight or lighter, and usually work up to no higher than ten-, fifteen-, and twenty-pound dumbbells. (If you are using machines, you will follow the specific machine-weight advice.)

The workout is similar to the next book I'll talk about, *Now or Never*, but with different exercises, and this is an excellent book to switch to if you are doing *Now or Never* and want to continue to build muscle but are getting bored with the exercises. Keep in mind, however, that if you switch to *Top Shape* you will have to add in a hips/buttocks routine from one of my other workouts, and that for women the thigh routine is not optional! (Many men feel that they don't want to use weights to exercise their legs since their lower body is rarely seen in public and they run or play a sport that, at least to some extent, exercises their legs. Therefore, I've made the lower-body workout optional for the men!)

NOW OR NEVER

Like *Top Shape*, *Now or Never* is a less intense workout than *Definition*, *The Fat-Burning Workout*, or *Bottoms Up!* But it allows you to develop more of a muscle base than any other workout yet discussed (except *Top Shape*, which allows an equal amount or more of muscle building).

The workout takes forty minutes if you shorten the thirty-second rests to fifteen seconds. Otherwise, it takes a full hour. You begin working with three-, five-, and ten-pound dumbbells and work your way up to ten-, fifteen-, and twenty-pound dumbbells—or higher, depending upon how much of a muscle base you wish to create.

Like *The Fat-Burning Workout*, *Bottoms Up!*, and *Top Shape*, the workout utilizes the modified pyramid system, where you add weight to each of three sets at the expense of a few repetitions.

Now or Never features a machine workout photographed at a fitness center using various machines. If you want to incorporate machines into your workout, you can use this book to get a clear idea about how to use them.

How will you know if it is time to switch to *Now or Never*? Take a hard look at your body and ask yourself if you need more of a muscle base. If your triceps have improved somewhat but are still slightly waving in the wind even after doing one of my other workouts, switch to *Now or Never*, at least for that body part, for six months to a year or more. If you are an older woman and you notice that after you have lost your excess body fat, your front thigh muscle is sagging and hanging over your knee, you should switch to the thigh workout in *Now or Never*. In fact, you would probably be doing yourself a real favor if you switched to *Now or Never* for your total body workout for at least six months to a year!

WEIGHT TRAINING MADE EASY: TRANSFORM YOUR BODY IN FOUR SIMPLE STEPS

This book does exactly what the title says it does: It makes things simple and brings you along step by step. Nothing is assumed; everything is explained clearly and simply. You are taken from workout level 1 (the easiest) through workout level 4, the most challenging. Each workout takes approximately twenty to thirty minutes, four to six days a week. The workouts include: Level 1: Learning the Moves; Level 2: Establishing a Muscle Base; Level 3: Sculpting and Defining the Muscles; and Level 4: The Finishing Touch. Each workout level requires a little more effort and a little more thinking, but the graduated levels are done in such a manner that by the time you reach level 4 you are truly an expert. In many ways, this book is four books in one, but much less intimidating than four books would be.

Weight Training Made Easy pulls the whole idea of weight training all together! Not only does it gently lead the reader along from one stage to the next in a nonintimidating way, but it also provides a clear, photographed explanation of how to substitute barbells and machines for dumbbells if you so desire. In addition, everything in that book is simplified, even the diet. I wrote the book because of popular demand. Many of my readers were writing and asking me to write one book that pulls it all together for them. This is the book!

Specialized Workouts

GUT BUSTERS

There is a special book I've written just for stomach work: *Gut Busters*. Although it is addressed to men, women do exactly the same workout. It contains the seven exercises most used by champion body-builders and, in fact, this is how most of them get their amazing mid-sections. If you are tired of doing the stomach work in the Bathing Suit Workout, or if you switch to another book but still want to bomb away at your stomach only with different exercises than are found in *The Bathing Suit Workout*, switch to *Gut Busters*.

Once you get used to the workout, it takes only fifteen minutes a day. Since no weights are used with the workout, you do not use the pyramid system or the modified pyramid system. You simply do fifteen to twenty-five repetitions per set of exercises, doing three sets for each body part with a fifteen-second rest between each set. It is very simple to follow.

BONE BUILDING BODY SHAPING WORKOUT

This is a specialized book featuring a routine that can be done in eight minutes a day for a minimum workout—up to thirty-two minutes a day for a maximum workout. It includes body-shaping and bone-building exercises specifically organized for women most interested in protecting themselves against future problems with fractures. The skeleton is featured and each bone being enhanced by each exercise is clearly shown, as well as each muscle that is being reshaped. The diet in the book is especially geared not only to weight loss, but also to calcium-rich foods. The workout gives tone and shape—and definition—all the while, building bone from every angle.

THE BOTTOMS UP WORKOUT: MIDDLE BODY VIDEO

There is yet another special stomach workout on video, *The Bottoms Up Workout: Middle Body*. It takes the stomach work from the book *Bottoms Up!* but greatly expands the workout, giving ten instead of six abdominal exercises and changing some of the exercises so that people with problem backs can also do them.

If you want to use *The Bottoms Up Workout: Middle Body* video, you can either use it to replace the stomach workout in the book you are using or you can alternate it with the stomach workout contained in the book!

Another way to use either of the specialized stomach workouts, *Gut Busters* or *The Bottoms Up Workout: Middle Body*, is to do one workout one day and the other workout the next day, six days a week and alternating days—one day *Gut Busters* and the next day *The Bottoms Up Workout: Middle Body*.

Finally, you can do the stomach workout contained in the book you are using, and on alternate days do either *Gut Busters* or *The Bottoms Up*

Workout: Middle Body, for a three-day routine, and then repeat the sequence. On the seventh day, give your stomach muscles a break from working out.

When Should You Change Workouts?

As a general rule, you should not switch workouts for about six weeks. However, the 12-Minute Total-Body Workout may be used as just a break-in to weight training or as a vacation for you, and you may want to use it for only a few weeks.

With all the other workouts, however, it's a good idea to allow six to twelve weeks to really see what the workout can do for you. If you like what you are seeing and want more of it, stick with your workout for another three months. You can even remain with a workout as long as a year or more, though it is really better to switch after about a year to shock your body into further development.

How to Decide Which Workout You Should Do Next

Your decision about which workout to do next will depend upon two things: what you see in the mirror and how much time and energy you have to invest.

Suppose, for example, you have been doing the Fat-Burning Workout along with the Bathing Suit Workout, but you feel that you need more muscle on your upper body and, in addition, you are bored with the Bathing Suit Workout. The ideal thing to do is to switch to workouts in *Bottoms Up!*, *Now or Never*, or *Top Shape*. Each of these workouts will give you more of a muscle base. In addition, both give a total-body workout, although *Bottoms Up!* gives more work for hips/butt, thighs, and stomach than does *Now or Never* or *Top Shape*.

Now let's take a different scenario. Suppose you took my advice in the earlier paragraphs of this book. You added *Bottoms Up!* to your Bathing Suit Workout for a total-body workout (leaving out hips/butt, thigh, and abdominal work from *Bottoms Up!*, of course, because you are already doing that with your Bathing Suit Workout). After a few months you look in the mirror and think, "I want more definition. Also, I want a shorter workout." Perfect. Switch to *Definition*. You'll get maximum cuts, burn more fat, and, in addition, you'll shorten your workout to fifteen minutes a day! If that workout is just a bit too intense and you have the extra five minutes to spare, instead go to *The Fat-Burning Workout* or *The College Dorm Workout*.

Now let's take a third scenario. Suppose you've been doing *Now or Never* because you've felt a need for more of a muscle base. But now you're burned out on working out and you really feel like taking a three-month vacation from it all. Don't do it. Instead, switch to *The 12-Minute Total-Body Workout*. As the title indicates, you'll only have to work out twelve minutes a day, but the return for your efforts will be worth hours a day because this workout will maintain your hard-earned muscles and when you are ready to go back to one of my longer workouts, you will not have to go through much muscle soreness—perhaps none at all. This workout provides enough of a challenge to your muscles to keep them "at the ready."

My Prescription: *If You Don't Want to Think about It*

If you want to make sure your body enjoys the benefit of a wide variety of exercise, pick any of my workouts, do it for three months, and then switch to another.

What order should you take? It won't matter in the long run. Over time, as long as you do all of my workouts, your body will have gorgeous muscles, sexy definition, and it will be tight, toned, and shaped to the hilt. It's inevitable. How so? In time, you would be taking advantage of all of the basic body-shaping principles invented by champion bodybuilders, techniques that, like the law of gravity, cannot fail to reshape and define your body over time.

In review, here is the list of my exercise books according to length of workout, from shortest to longest, from least muscle building to most muscle building:

1. *The 12-Minute Total Body Workout*—Twelve minutes every day

2. *Definition*—Fifteen minutes six days a week, or thirty minutes three days a week

3. *The College Dorm Workout*—Twenty minutes five to six days a week

4. *The Fat-Burning Workout*—Twenty minutes four to six days a week

5. *Bottoms Up!*—Twenty to thirty minutes four to six days a week

6. *Top Shape*—Thirty to forty minutes four to six days a week

7. *Now or Never*—Forty to sixty minutes four to six days a week

8. *Weight Training Made Easy*—Twelve to thirty minutes four to seven days a week (depending upon which of the four levels you are doing)

Specialized Workouts

9. *Gut Busters*—Fifteen minutes four to six days a week

10. *Bone Building Body Shaping Workout*—Eight to thirty-two minutes two to six days a week

11. *The Bottoms Up Workout: Middle Body* (Video)—Twenty to thirty minutes three to six days a week

Note: Books are available in all major bookstores. Videos can be ordered through me. See pp. 199–200 for further details.

Taking Time Off from Working Out with Weights

The most time you should take off is one week every six months to a year. This adds up to a total of no more than two weeks off a year from working out with weights. Why take a break at all? The human body is not much different from the human mind when it comes to boredom. It simply needs a change! If you tried never to take time off from working out with weights, after a while your body would rebel and would refuse to cooperate with you. Every workout would become a struggle. You would have to fight yourself with each repetition. You'd be tempted to quit in the middle of a workout.

The bottom line is, you can't fool mother nature. So don't try to behave as if your body were a machine. It's not. It's human, and made of flesh and bone. So think ahead and take time off—at least one week a year. Don't worry. You don't have to vegetate completely during that time. You can still walk, engage in sports, or even do a favorite aerobic activity. Just stay away from the weights for a week.

The Lifetime Guarantee

If you make up your mind to incorporate a weight-training workout into your daily routine (well, at least four days a week) and, better, if you do aerobics at least three times a week in addition (this will give you an exercise regimen for each day of the week), I promise that even if you do overeat and gain some weight, you will never go back to being as out of shape as you were before you started. In addition, I promise that it will be relatively easy to get back in shape once you start again. All you will have to do is to follow, once again, the low-fat eating plan in any of my fitness books, or a doctor-approved, low-fat, balanced diet of your own choosing.

Why does this work? Your hard-earned muscles and the beautiful definition will be there waiting for you under the fat, whereas had you completely stopped working out, your muscles would have slowly atrophied. You would now have soft flab under the fat, and would have double the trouble getting back in shape.

But even if you did the wrong thing and stopped working out in addition to pigging out, there's good news. Muscles remember! Yes, every muscle you build is like putting muscle in the permanent memory bank. Once you start working out again, it takes only one third the time it took you originally to get the muscles. In other words, say you worked out for a year and got in shape. Then you stopped working out for a year. It takes only four months to get back what it took you a year to get the first time. (And by the way, it takes as long as you took to get the muscles to lose them. In other words, it takes a whole year to lose muscles you built for a year, two years to lose all the muscles you build after working out for two years, and so on.)

So the bottom line is that you've got nothing to lose and everything to gain from working out with weights—even if you do let yourself go. But the key is not to let yourself go. Incorporate working out into your daily life plan for now and forever!

A Final Note

If you wish to write me to make a comment or ask a question or to send me your "before-and-after"s, please include a stamped, self-addressed envelope and I will personally reply. See p. 199 for address.

News Flash

I'm having a special cruise for fun and fitness. If you're interested, call Gotta Go Cruises at the toll free number: 888-446-8824.

BIBLIOGRAPHY

Videos by Joyce Vedral

Vedral, Joyce. *The Bottoms Up Workout: Upper Body*. New York: Good Times Video, 1995. $14.98. (See below to order.)

Vedral, Joyce. *The Bottoms Up Workout: Middle Body*. New York: Good Times Video, 1995. $14.98. (See below to order.)

Vedral, Joyce. *The Bottoms Up Workout: Lower Body*. New York: Good Times Video, 1995. $14.98. (See below to order.) Note: $39.98 if you buy all three.

Vedral, Joyce. *The Fat-Burning Workout: Volume I*. Regular Workout. (20 minutes a day). New York: Time-Life Video, 1993. $21.98. (See below to order.)

Vedral, Joyce. *The Fat-Burning Workout: Volume II*. Intensity and Insanity Workout. (40 minutes a day). New York: Time-Life Video, 1993. $21.98. (See below to order.)

To order, add $3.95 for each item for shipping and handling. Send a check or money order to:

Joyce L. Vedral
P.O. Box 7433
Wantagh, NY 11793-7433

Note: if you order the Bottoms Up Series, all three, you need send only $3.95. Also, if you order Volumes II and III of *The Fat Burning Workout*, you need send only $3.95.

INDEX

Page numbers of illustrations appear in italics

Abdominals: rectus abdominal, external, oblique, and internal oblique, 2, *41*, 42–43
 alternating routines for, 193–94
 bent-knee sewn lift, 74, *75*
 Bottoms Up Workout: Middle Body (video) for, 193
 ceiling oblique reach, 104, *105*
 ceiling sewn lift, 92, *93*
 exercise routines, frequency, 43–44
 Gut Busters workout for, 192–93
 knee-in, 110, *110*
 knee-raised crunch
 knee-raised oblique crunch, 68, *69*
 leg raise, 122, *123*
 regular bathing suit workout, exercises for, 52
 side oblique crunch, 86, *87*
 sit-up, 116, *117*
 "six pack," 42
 toe-reach crunch, 98, *99*
Adductor muscle. *See* Machines; Thighs
Aerobic dance, 155–56
Aerobic exercise. *See* Exercise, aerobic
Age, and reshaping body, 45
Alcohol, 136
Arms, workout for, 184

Back problems, modifying exercises, 51, 58
Basal metabolism, 21
Before and After
 Anita, 25–26, *26*
 Chris, 24–25, *24*
 Ivonne, 23–24, *24*
 Joyce, *22*, 23
 Kelley, 28, *28*, 29
 Michelle, 26–27, *27*

you, 29, *29*
Bent-knee deadlift, 114, *115*
Bent-knee sewn lift, 74, *75*
Bicycle riding (stationary or moving at a moderate pace), 159–60
Bone Building Body Shaping Workout (Vedral), 138, 193, 196
Bone density
 Bone Building Body Shaping Workout for, 193
 calcium for, 138
 Joyce's, 138, 181
 working out with weights, 181
Bottoms Up! (Vedral), 26, 29, 74, 92, 184, 185, 189–90, 194, 195, 196
 videos available, 190
Bottoms Up Workout: Lower Body (video), 190
Bottoms Up Workout: Middle Body (video), 173, 174, 190
Bottoms Up Workout: Upper Body (video), 190
Box aerobics (boxercise), 153–54
Breathing, during exercise, 33–34
Buttocks, 23. *See also* Hips/buttocks

Caffeine, 136
Calcium, 137–38
 Bone Building Body Shaping Workout and, 193
 food sources, 138
Calories
 burned per hour, resting, 21
 dietary fat versus carbohydrate and protein, 12
 how to know you're not consuming too many, 136
 one pound of body fat and, 12, 165
Calves, workout, 184

Carbohydrates, 10, 131–35
    hindering fat burning, 132, 134
    limited complex, 132–33
    percentage recommended, 127
    simple (fruit), 134
    sugar and refined, 18, 132
    unlimited complex (vegetables), 133–34
Ceiling sewn lift, 92, *93*
Cellulite, 3–4, 46
    liposuction and, 171
Chair position firmer, 78, *79*
Cheese, fat content, 17
    low-fat, 17
Chest exercises, 184
Cholesterol, 14
    bad (LDL), 14–15
    good (HDL), 14–15
    index, 15
College Dorm Workout (Vedral), 189, 194, 195
Complete Book of Cosmetic Surgery, The, 177
Concentration (on muscle), 36
Continual pressure (on muscle), 36
Cosmetic surgery, 167–79
    areas exercise cannot help, 168
    face, eyes, and neck, 168
    finding a surgeon, 177–78
    full and mini tummy tucks, 172–75
    hip, thigh, and butt lifts, 175–77
    liposuction, 168–72
    making the decision, 177
    working out and, 167, 179
Cross-country skiing, 152–53

Dairy foods, 131, 134, 135
    as calcium source, 138
Dancing
    aerobic, 155–56
    quick pace, 160–61
Definition (of muscle), 37
Definition (Vedral), 23, 26, 29, 184, 185, 187,
    194, 195
Density (of muscle), 37–38
Desserts, 131, 134
Diet (weight loss and maintenance), 5, 7, 182
    alcohol, 136
    balanced low-fat diet, percentages daily,
        127
    basic food rules, 141
    caffeine, 136
    calcium, 137–38
    carbohydrates, 10, 127, 131–35
    dairy, 131, 134, 135
    desserts, 131, 134

fat, 10, 11, 14, 15, 127
fiber, 135
food pyramid, USDA, 128, *128*
forbidden foods, 15–17
free eating day, 140–41
frequency of eating, 139
meal plans, 141–43
percentage versus grams of fat, 13
pizza, 18
protein, 10, 127, 129–31
salt or sodium, 137
sugar and refined carbohydrates, 18, 134
water, 138–39
Dynamic tension, 36

Eat to Trim (Vedral), 11, 143
Equipment for exercises, 4, 39–40
    barbell, 84, 90, 102, 114
    dumbbell, 40, 51, 52, 68, 74, 80, 86, 92,
        96, 104, 108, 110, 116
Essential fatty acids, 11
Exercise, aerobic, 6–7, 35–36, 57, 154–65
    bicycle riding (stationary or moving at a
        moderate pace), 159–60
    box aerobics (boxercise), 153–54
    breaking in, new activity, 150–51
    breaking in, general, for newcomers,
        149–50
    cross-country skiing, 152–53
    daily, at home or office, 164–65
    dancing at a quick pace (freestyle or
        country/western), 160–61
    Definition workout as, 187
    fat-burning and, 145, 161, 164
    fat-burning exercise chart, 147
    frequency of workouts, 148
    high-impact, 156
    hiking (hills), 157–58
    household activities, 163–64
    jogging at a slow pace, 158–59
    low-impact (aerobic dance), 155–56
    maximum pulse rate, figuring, 35–36,
        146–47
    NordicTrack and other machines, 156
    pool aerobics and water walking, 160
    racewalking, 157
    rope-jumping, 155
    rowing machine, 158
    running (outdoors or treadmill), 151–52
    sports, 161–63
    stair-stepping, 154–55
    step aerobics, 154
    swimming, 153

trampoline jumping, 156–57

walking at a quick pace, 161

weight-training/bathing suit workout and, 149

workout length (of time), 148

Exercise, Bathing Suit Workout, 31

aerobic, eliminating rests to make, 57

aerobics, do before or after, 149

attitude toward exercise, 49

breaking in gently, 59–60

changing routines and workouts, 185, 194, 195

choosing workouts, 194–95

details concerning muscles, 37–39

emergency ten, 2

how to do, 51–62

information (definitions of terms), 31–35

instructions, how to use, 58–58

intensity, reducing, 57

iron woman workout, 55

magic seven (seven tri-sets of regular workout), 2, 52

maintaining, 183

plans: fitting it into your real-life, 43–44

review of exercises, 125

steel woman workout, 55

technique information, 35–37

time required for, 3, 4–5

timing of, during day, 44

titanium woman workout, 56

tri-set, 2–3, 51, 52–54

what results to expect, 7

Exercise devices, 45

Exercise, workouts for rest of body, 184–85

Fast food restaurant dishes

beef products, 16

chicken, 16

croissant dishes, 16

dessert products, 16

fish, 16

hamburgers, 16

hidden in salad and pasta, 17

low-fat alternatives, 17

Mexican food, 16

pizza, 18

potato dishes, 16

Fat, body

brown, 20

-burning activities, 48, 145–65

-burning chart, 147

calories to cause one pound, 12, 165

carbohydrates that hinder burning, 132, 134

dietary fat and, 12

heredity and, 46

location of, 12, 19

measurement of, 47–48

muscle to burn, 21

percentage, 19, 47–48

-remover creams, 45

water intake and, 18

weight, appearance, and, 20

Fat-Burning Workout, The (Vedral), 26, 28, 29, 184, 187–88, 194, 195

videos available, 188

Fat, dietary

American diet, 10

calories in one gram, 12

daily percent versus grams, 13

digesting, 12

foods, high fat, 15–17

foods, surprising amounts in, 11

hidden fat content, 17

need in diet, 11

"98 percent fat free," 13

percentage needed in diet, 10, 127

polyunsaturated, 14

sources, 131

too little in diet, 11

trans fatty acids, 14

Fear of failure, 47

Fiber, 135

Floor feather kick-up, 88, *89*

Food. *See also* Carbohydrates; Dairy; Diet; Fast food restaurants; Fat, dietary; Fruit; Protein; Vegetables

components of, 10

label, "98% fat free," 13

pyramid, USDA, 128, *128*

Free eating day, 140–41

Fruit, 133–34. *See also* Carbohydrates, simple

alcohol as substitute for, 136

juice, 134

Giant set, 32, 187, 189

Gotta Go Cruises, 197

Gut Busters (Vedral), 29, 173, 174, 189, 192–93, 196

Hack squat, 108, *109*

Hamstrings. *See* Thighs

Hiking (hills), 157–58

Hip, thigh, and butt lifts (cosmetic surgery procedures), 175–77

Hip, thigh, and butt lifts (continued)
  disappointment with and scarring, 177
  do you really need it, 176
  how it is performed, 175
  what it can and cannot do, 176
Hips/buttocks: gluteus maximus, gluteus
    medius, gluteus minimus, 2, 40, *41*, 42
  exercise routines, frequency, 43–44
  floor feather kick-up, 88, *89*
  lower butt crunch, 76, 77
  lower butt curl, 70, *71*
  lower butt side kick, 82, *83*
  lying butt lift, 94, *95*
  one-leg prone butt lift, 100, *101*
  regular bathing suit workout, exercises for,
    52
  reverse-lunge lift, 112, *112*
  saddlebag stripper, 64, *65*
  standing butt squeeze, 106, *106*
  straight leg kick-up, 118, *119*
  weights, optional, 106, 110
Household activities, aerobic aspect of,
    163–64

Intensity (of exercise), 36
Iron woman workout, 55
Isometric pressure, 36

Jogging at a slow pace, 158–59

Knee-in, 110, *110*
Knee problems, modifying exercises, 51, 58
Knee-raised oblique crunch, 68, *69*

Leg curl, 72, *73*
Leg raise, 122, *123*
Leg routine. *See* Thighs
Liposuction, 168–72
  cellulite and, 171
  discoloration of skin after, 172
  do you really need it, 169–70
  gaining weight after, 170–71
  how it is performed, 169
  ideal time for, 170
  lift (surgical) needed after, 171
  what it can and cannot do, 170
Liptase, 132
*Look In, Look Up, Look Out: Be the Person You
    Were Meant to Be* (Vedral), 21
Lower butt crunch, 76, 77
Lower butt curl, 70, *71*
Lower butt side kick, 82, *83*
Low-impact aerobics (aerobic dance), 155–56

Lying butt lift, 94, *95*
Lying inner thigh lift, 66, *67*

Machines (gym), using for workouts, 59
  butt-curl, 70, 76
  crunch machine, 80
  hip abductor, 64
  hip adductor, 66
  hips/buttocks, 78, 88, 94, 100, 112, 118
  leg-curl, 72
  leg-press, 90
  Now or Never workout and, 191
  Roman chair, 122
  rotary butt, 82
  rotary torso, 68, 86
  squat, 84
  Top Shape workout and, 190
Macronutrients, 10
Meal plans, 141–43
Micronutrients, 10
Minerals, 10
Motivation, 21
Muscle, 21
  anatomy of, used in Bathing Suit Workout,
    40–43, *41*
  atrophy of, 43
  concentration, 36
  continual pressure on, 36
  definition, 37
  density, 37–38
  dynamic tension on, 36, 189
  fat-burning by, 48, 181
  flexed, 34
  forty-eight hour recovery principle, 38
  injury, 39
  isolation, 35
  isometric pressure on, 36, 189
  mass, 37
  soreness, 39
  split-routine, 38, 43
  sticking points, 38–39
  stretched, 34
  symmetry, 38
  tears, 39
  upper-body, and swimming, 153
Muscularity, 37

NordicTrack and other machines, 156
Now or Never (Vedral), 176, 191–92, 194, 195

Obesity and excess weight
  American, 9
  Bathing Suit Workout and, 51

breaking in gently to do exercises, 60–61
emotional issue, 182
reducing intensity and starting slowly, 57–58
One-leg prone butt lift, 100, *101*
Osteoporosis, preventing, 181
Bone Building Body Shaping Workout for, 193

Pizza, 18
Plateau, 35
Pool aerobics and water walking, 160
Poultry, skinless, 130
Pritikin Longevity Center, 10
Progression, 35
Protein, 129–31
grams per pound of body weight, 129
percentage recommended, 127, 129
sources of low-fat, 130–31
Pyramid system
Bathing Suit Workout and, 51, 52
Bottoms Up! workout and, 190
Definition workout and, 187, 188
Fat-Burning Workout and, 188
modified, 32–33, 68, 80, 188, 190, 191
Top Shape workout and, 191
true or regular, 32–33, 187, 188

Racewalking, 157
Repetitions, 31, 52, 63
Rests, 33, 57
Reverse-lunge lift, 112, *112*
Rope-jumping, 155
Routine, 34
Rowing machine, 158
Running (outdoors or treadmill), 151–52

Saddlebag stripper, 64, *65*
Salt or sodium, 137
Set, 31
giant, 32, 187, 189
speed, 32
speed supersets, 187
super or "twin," 184, 190
Shoulders, workout for, 184
Side oblique crunch, 86, *87*
Sissy squat, 120, *121*
Sit-up, 116, *117*
Skinny-fat, 23
Soreness, 39
Speed sets, 32
Speed supersets, 187
Split-routine, 38, 43

Sports, 161–63
calorie chart, 162–63
Spot-reducing versus spot-reshaping, 46–47
Stair
climbing, 165
-stepping machine, 48–49, 154–55
Standing butt squeeze, 106, *106*
Steel woman workout, 55
Step aerobics, 154
Sticking points, 38–39
Stomach. *See* Abdominals
Straddle squat, 84, *85*
Stretching, 53
Sugar and refined carbohydrates, 18, 132
Superset, 32, 184, 190
speed, 32
Swimming, 153
pool aerobics and water walking, 160

Target date, 35
Telephone talking, activity during, 164
Thighs: quadriceps, adductor, and biceps femoris or hamstrings, 2, *41*, 42
bent-knee deadlift, 114, *115*
chair position firmer, 78, *79*
exercise routines, frequency, 43–44
front squat, 90, *91*
hack squat, 108, *109*
leg curl,,72, *73*
lifting through exercise versus surgery, 176
lunge, 96, *97*
lying inner thigh lift, 66, *67*, 68
regular bathing suit workout, exercises for, 53
sagging over knee problem, 4
saddlebags (outer thigh), 40, *41*, 42
sissy squat, 120, *121*
squat (regular), 102, *103*
straddle squat, 84, *85*
weights for exercises, 32, 33, 39, 49, 52, 74, 80, 84, 86, 90, 96, 98, 102, 104, 108, 110, 114, 116
Titanium woman workout, 56
Toe-reach crunch, 98, *99*
Toning, 5–6
Top Shape (Vedral), 29, 176, 190–91, 194, 195
Trampoline jumping, 156–57
Treadmill, exercising on, 152
Tri-set, 2–3, 32, 51, 52
how they work, 53–53
seven of regular Bathing Suit Workout, 52
speed, 32

Tummy tuck, full, 172–73
  do you really need it, 172–73
  how performed (and scar left), 172
  gaining weight after, 173
  ideal time to get, 173
  what it can and cannot do, 173
Tummy tuck, mini, 174–75
  do you really need it, 174
  how performed and scar left, 174
  ideal time to get, 175
  what it can and cannot do, 175
12-Minute Total-Body Workout, The (Vedral),
  186, 195
Twin set 184, 190

Vedral, Marthe, *126*
Vegetables, 133. *See also* Carbohydrates,
  unlimited complex
Visualization, 36
  unconscious mind and, 36–37
Vitamins, 10

Walking
  after a meal, 164
  dog, 165
  parking car and, 165
  quick pace, 161
Water (dietary), 10, 138–39
  fat-burning and, 18
  intake per day, 19, 139
  pills, 46
Water exercise (pool aerobics and water
  walking), 160

Weight gain
  changing thinking about, 182–83
  emotional issue of, 182
Weight loss. *See also* Calories; Diet
  exercise before dieting, 48
  working out as lifestyle, 183
Weights, 34
  barbell use during Bathing Suit Workout,
    84, 90, 102, 114
  Bottoms Up! workout and, 190
  College Dorm Workout and, 190
  Definition workout and, 187
  dumbbell use during Bathing Suit Workout,
    32, 33, 39, 40, 49, 51, 52, 68, 74, 80,
    92, 96, 104, 108, 110, 116
  Fat-Burning Workout and, 188
  lifetime guarantee, 196–97
  lifting sagging skin with versus surgery,
    176
  Now or Never workout and, 191–92
  osteoporosis prevention and, 181
  taking time off from working, 196
  Top Shape workout and, 190–91
  12-Minute Total-Body Workout and, 186
  weightbelt, 120
  Weight Training Made Easy workout and,
    192
Weight Training Made Easy (Vedral), 185, 186,
  192, 196
Workout, 34. *See* Exercise, Bathing Suit
  Workout

ABOUT THE AUTHOR

We'll never forget the day in 1991, when Joyce Vedral appeared on the *Sally Jessy Raphael Show*. It was a quiet July morning and Joyce had been invited on the program to promote her new book, *The Fat-Burning Workout*. With a built-in flair for the dramatic, Joyce decided to appear on camera in a provocative gold bikini that showed off her toned, enviable forty-eight-year-old figure to best effect.

If we told you that all hell broke loose a mere five minutes into the broadcast, it wouldn't begin to describe the pandemonium that followed as viewers all over the country raced out to find copies of Joyce's workout. "If she can do it, I can do it too," they cried to bookstore owners, the Warner switchboard, and to anyone who would listen. In no time, Joyce was a recognized fitness guru, well on her way to the *New York Times* bestseller list.

If anyone ever tells you that lightning does not strike twice, don't believe them. Joyce did it again. She appeared on the *Montel Williams Show* and had an even greater reaction to her book *Bottoms Up!* For the week of January 1, 1994, her book beat all books in print in America, including books by Howard Stern, Rush Limbaugh, and Michael Crichton—making number one on the *USA Today* list for that week. That same book, *Bottoms Up!*, reached number one on the *New York Times* bestseller list.

Today, at a fit and classy fifty-five, Joyce's fitness library combines for an in-print total of well over one million copies. The reason books like *Bottoms Up! Top Shape, Definition, Gutbusters, The 12-Minute Total-Body Workout, Now or Never, Eat to Trim,* and *Weight Training Made Easy* have sold so well is simple: They achieve the promised results.

But there's another reason for Joyce's success: Joyce, with her trademark upbeat voice, is a real person who convinces people in lectures and on television shows all over the country that "if I can do it, so can you." She isn't shy about the before picture of herself, fat at twenty-six, nor is she afraid to poke fun at her "bad genetics." "I come from a Russian heritage," she says. "My whole family look like boxes on wheels."

When Joyce gives a lecture, people are mesmerized. She has a way of relating to an audience as if she knows each and every one personally, and a gift for getting right down to the level of each eager listener. In the words of Paul Adamo of The Learning Annex in New York City, "In all the years of my having lecturers I have never seen anything like this in my life. She arrests the audience and keeps each and every one of them in the palm of her hand throughout. People walk away with love in their eyes. No one can have a Joyce Vedral 'experience' without being touched."

Joyce is a frequent guest on *Oprah*, the *Today* show, *Sally Jessy Raphael*, and CNN, and has been written up in the *New York Times*, the *Daily News*, and the *Post*. She is a sought-after speaker in women's groups, fitness centers, and shopping malls across the country.

Perhaps what makes Joyce most interesting is her unusual background. Unlike so many other fitness experts who are one-dimensional, Joyce earned her Ph.D. in English literature from New York University. Her knowledge of fitness came after years of teaching high school and college English, getting "fat and out of shape," and by luck, landing freelance assignments to *Muscle and Fitness* and *Shape* magazines, where she became acquainted with the techniques that now fill her books and lectures. Joyce says, "My mission is to help others who lead busy lives and are interested in getting healthy and in shape in minutes rather than hours a day."

Always a women's advocate, and concerned with women's issues, Joyce is, in addition, the author of *Bone-Building Body-Shaping Workout* and the international best-seller, with Warner Books, *Get Rid of Him!*, a book that helps women build their self-esteem, discover their inner strength, and move on when it's time—and to find the right man—and her new self-help book, *Look In, Look Up, Look Out!*

APPENDIX

THE BATHING SUIT WORKOUT
Tear-Out Wall Chart

Once you learn the Bathing Suit Workout, you can use the convenient tear-out wall chart on the following pages. If you paste the pages together, you will have an overview of the entire workout in the order in which it is done.

TRI-SET #1

HIPS/BUTTOCKS: SADDLEBAG STRIPPER

START

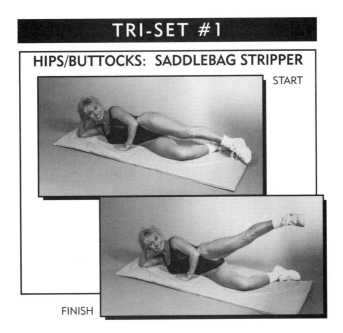

FINISH

THIGHS: LYING INNER THIGH LIFT

START

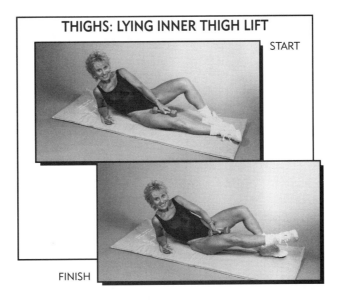

FINISH

ABDOMINALS: KNEE-RAISED OBLIQUE CRUNCH

START

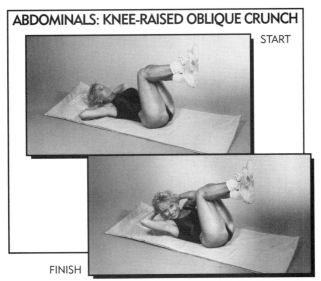

FINISH

TRI-SET #2

HIPS/BUTTOCKS: LOWER BUTT CURL

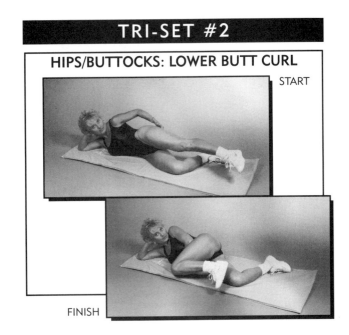

START

FINISH

THIGHS: LEG CURL

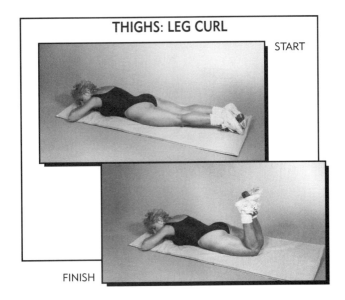

START

FINISH

ABDOMINALS: BENT-KNEE SEWN LIFT

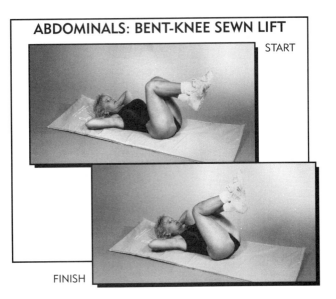

START

FINISH

TRI-SET #3

HIPS/BUTTOCKS: LOWER BUTT CRUNCH

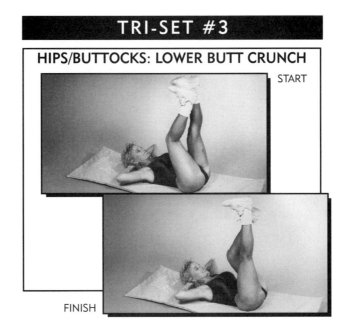

START

FINISH

THIGHS: CHAIR POSITION FIRMER

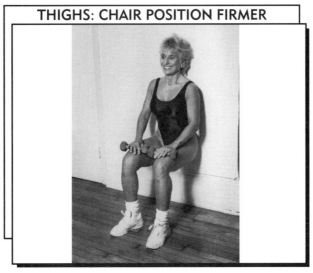

START   FINISH

ABDOMINALS: KNEE-RAISED CRUNCH

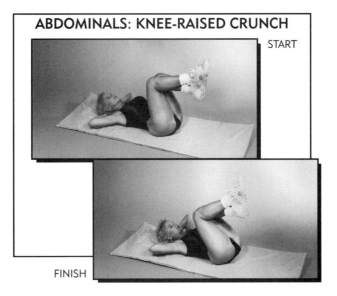

START

FINISH

TRI-SET #4

HIPS/BUTTOCKS: LOWER BUTT SIDE KICK

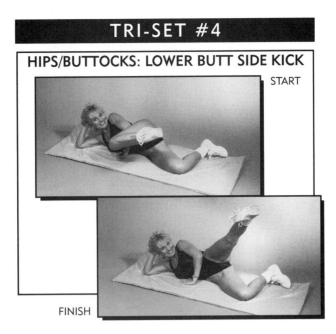

START

FINISH

THIGHS: STRADDLE SQUAT

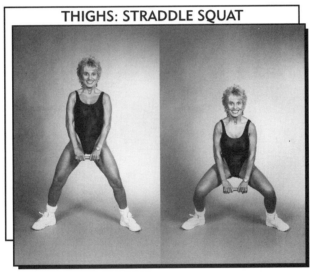

START FINISH

ABDOMINALS: SIDE OBLIQUE CRUNCH

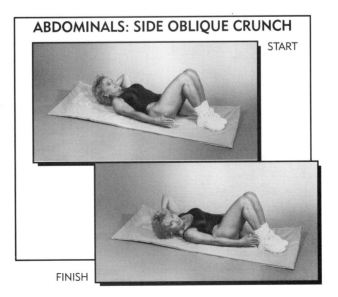

START

FINISH

TRI-SET #5

HIPS/BUTTOCKS: FLOOR FEATHER KICK-UP

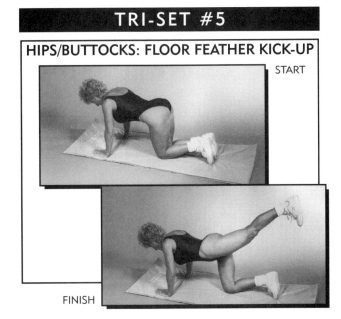

START

FINISH

THIGHS: FRONT SQUAT

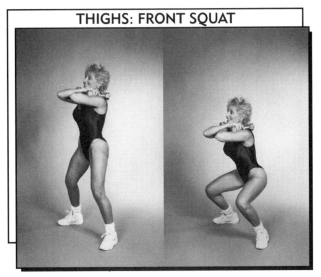

START   FINISH

ABDOMINALS: CEILING SEWN LIFT

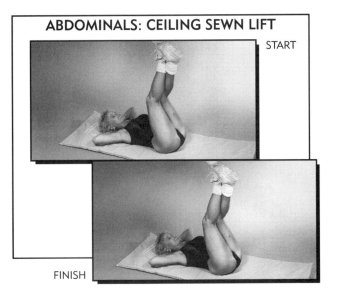

START

FINISH

TRI-SET #6

HIPS/BUTTOCKS: LYING BUTT LIFT

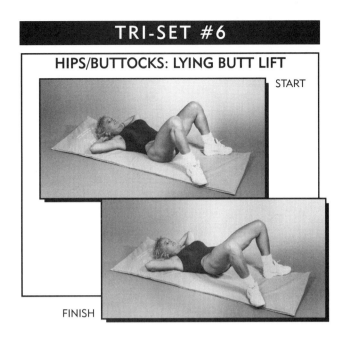

START

FINISH

THIGHS: LUNGE

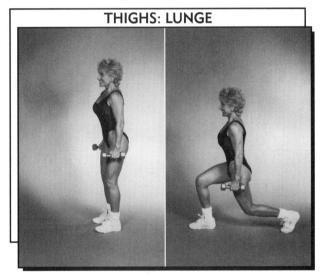

START   FINISH

ABDOMINALS: TOE-REACH CRUNCH

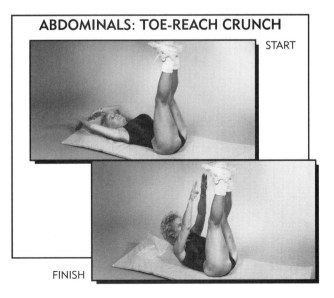

START

FINISH

TRI-SET #7

HIPS/BUTTOCKS: ONE-LEG PRONE BUTT LIFT

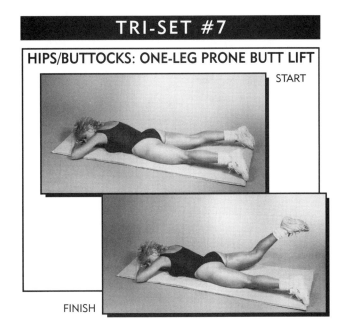

START

FINISH

THIGHS: REGULAR SQUAT

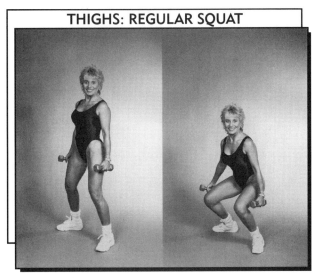

START   FINISH

ABDOMINALS: CEILING OBLIQUE REACH

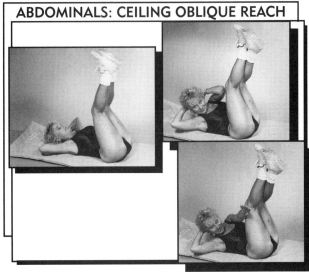

START   FINISH

TRI-SET #8

HIPS/BUTTOCKS: STANDING BUTT SQUEEZE

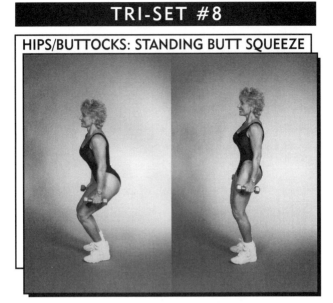

START   FINISH

THIGHS: HACK SQUAT

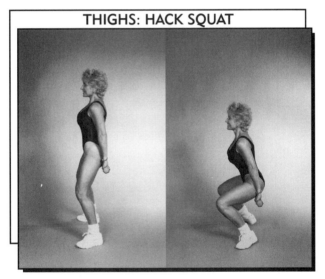

START   FINISH

ABDOMINALS: KNEE-IN

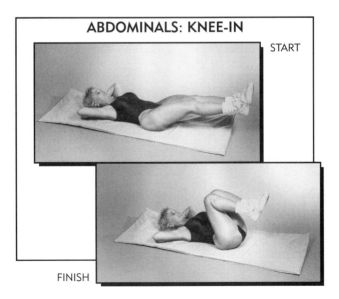

START

FINISH

TRI-SET #9

HIPS/BUTTOCKS: REVERSE LUNGE LIFT

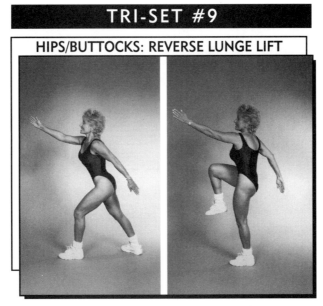

START   FINISH

THIGHS: BENT-KNEE DEADLIFT

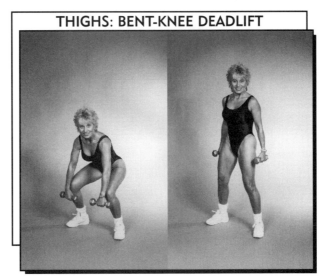

START   FINISH

ABDOMINALS: SIT-UP

START

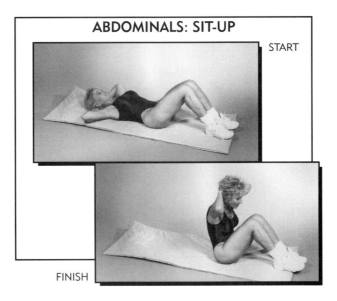

FINISH

TRI-SET #10

HIPS/BUTTOCKS: STRAIGHT-LEG KICK-UP

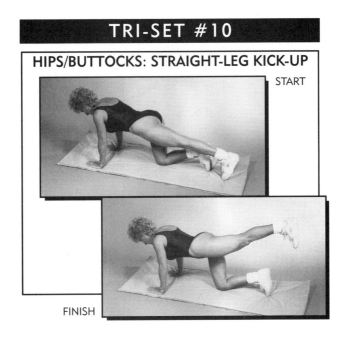

START

FINISH

THIGHS: SISSY SQUAT

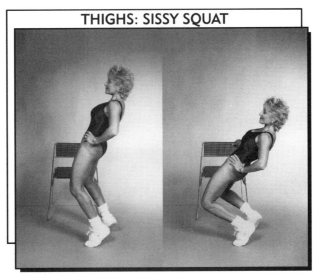

START   FINISH

ABDOMINALS: LEG RAISE

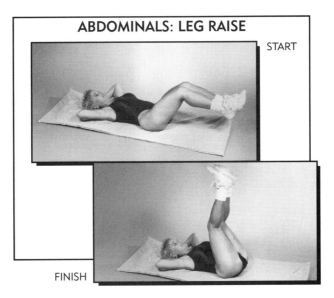

START

FINISH